El
Cl
HANDBOOK

B. Anderson

P. Shapiro

VAN NOSTRAND REINHOLD COMPANY
NEW YORK CINCINNATI TORONTO LONDON MELBOURNE

First published in paperback in 1982
Copyright © 1979 by Delmar Publishers Inc.
Library of Congress Catalog Card Number 78-10473
ISBN 0-442-20979-7

All rights reserved. No part of this work covered by the copyright hereon
may be reproduced or used in any form or by any means—graphic,
electronic, or mechanical, including photocopying, recording, taping, or
information storage and retrieval systems—without written permission of the
publisher.
Printed in the United States of America

Van Nostrand Reinhold Company Inc.
135 West 50th Street New York, NY 10020

Van Nostrand Reinhold Publishing
1410 Birchmount Road, Scarborough, Ontario M1P 2E7

Van Nostrand Reinhold Australia Pty. Ltd.
480 Latrobe Street, Melbourne, Victoria 3000, Australia

Van Nostrand Reinhold Company Ltd.
Molly Millars Lane, Wokingham, Berkshire, England RG11 2PY

Cloth edition published 1979 by Van Nostrand Reinhold Company Inc.

16 15 14 13 12 11 10 9 8 7 6 5 4 3 2 1

The purpose of this book is to inform — and to supplement formal instruction. It is not intended to be a self-instructional or do-it-yourself text. Neither is it meant to replace medical supervision of childbirth.

Childbirth is a natural phenomenon that is occurring every minute of every day. Elective home births are becoming more prevalent and unscheduled deliveries outside the hospital environment are not infrequent. This handbook was written to give the emergency medical technician, policeman, firefighter, and any other person in attendance, an understanding of the labor and delivery experience. In this way the individual will be better prepared to give assistance to the expectant mother and her baby until medical help is available. It is suggested that the glossary at the end of the text be used when an unfamiliar term is encountered. Many illustrations reinforce and clarify the topics being discussed.

The authors are well qualified to write on the subject of childbirth, having had combined experience and education in obstetrical nursing over a course of several years. Barbara Anderson is the author of *Obstetrics for the Nurse*. She is a graduate of St. Mary's Hospital in Waterbury Connecticut and Chaminade University in Honolulu. She has held several administrative positions and served as consultant for state and local organizations. Mrs. Anderson is assistant administrator at the Kaiser Medical Center in Honolulu, Hawaii. In addition to administrative duties, she teaches emergency childbirth to airline personnel and Emergency Medical Trainees.

Pamela Shapiro is a graduate of California State University. She received certification as a Childbirth Educator from the International Childbirth Education Association and has received additional training in the use of Lamaze techniques. Mrs. Shapiro teaches parent education classes and is associated with the Childbirth Education Association of Seattle. As instructor, she has conducted teacher-training workshops in addition to classes designed to prepare expectant couples for childbirth.

Acknowledgments

The authors wish to acknowledge the contribution of the Childbirth Education Association of Seattle for the sharing of the Lamaze concepts and techniques, and to the men in the Wailupe Fire Station, the Honolulu Police Department, and the City and County of Honolulu for the photographs they submitted.

The authors also wish to acknowledge their indebtedness to Marion Li who typed the original draft from handwritten material . . . to Jean Seo, R.N. for her professional expertise . . . to Jim Leonard for the beautiful pictures of his firstborn . . . to George Monlux, M.D., Chief of Emergency Medicine, for his help and knowledge of the Emergency Medical Technician's role in medicine.

The authors are most grateful to the publisher and editors, and in particular to Angela Emmi for her expert guidance and editing throughout the time span of writing and rewriting the final copy. Appreciation is also extended to Ruth Saur and Hazel Kozakiewicz for their contributions.

We wish to express a particular debt of gratitude to Mike Shapiro for his understanding and many contributions, and to Walter Fuller for his encouragement in the preparation of this book.

Medical illustrations by Mary Ann Kozakiewicz

Contents

BEFORE CHILDBIRTH

1. The Female Reproductive System.... 1
2. Ovulation and Menstruation 15
3. The Male Reproductive System...... 23
4. The Beginning of Life 33
5. Prenatal Development............. 43

LABOR AND DELIVERY

6. Understanding Labor............... 59
7. Emergency Delivery 84
8. Complications and Unusual Deliveries..................... 113

AFTER CHILDBIRTH

9. Postnatal Care of the Mother and New Baby.................. 149
10. Arriving at the Hospital............ 157

APPENDIX

A-1 List of Emergency Supplies......... 162
A-2 Lamaze Techniques................ 163
A-3 Ways to Hold an Infant............ 176
A-4 Terms Related to Childbirth 178
A-5 Optional Test and Answers 187

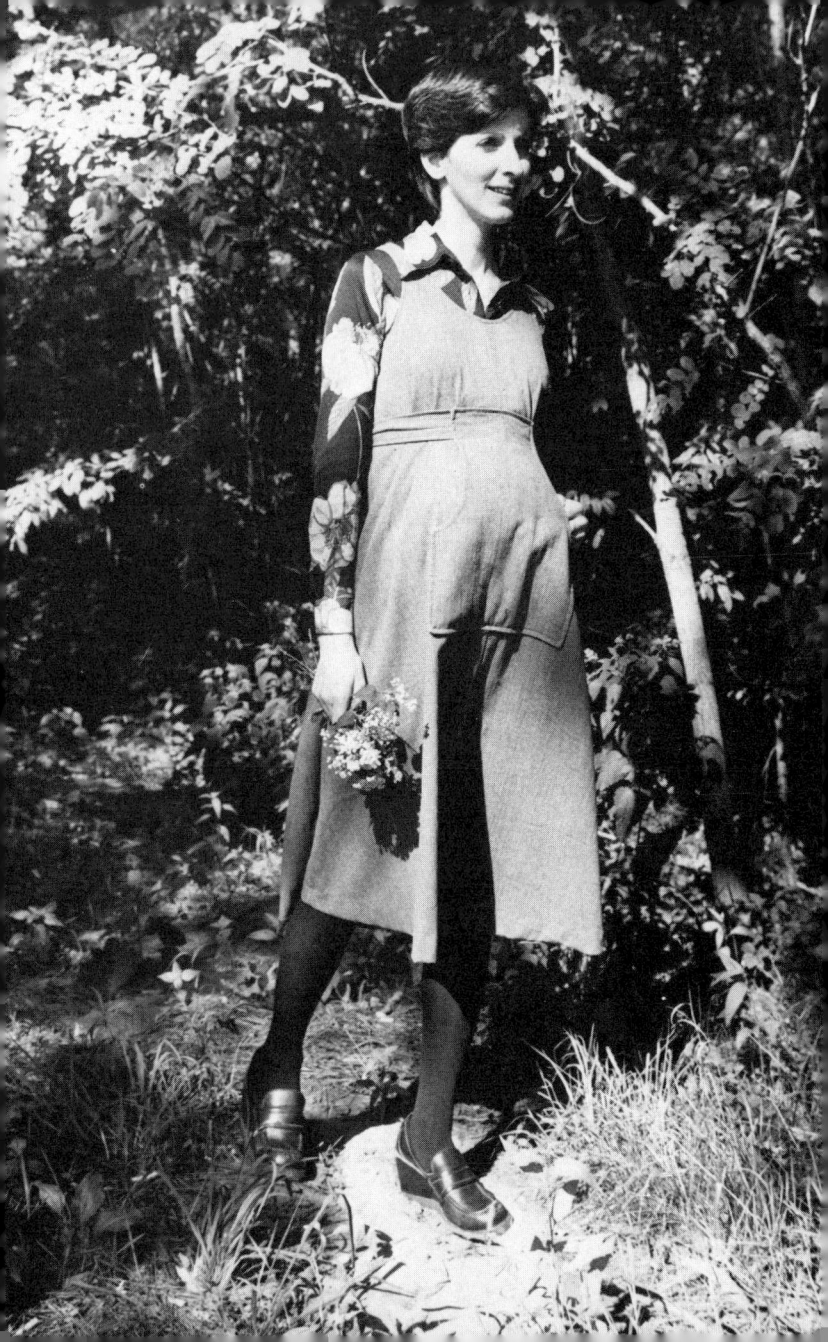

SECTION 1
BEFORE CHILDBIRTH

-1-
The Female Reproductive System

Human reproduction is the process by which a man and a woman create a new individual. An understanding of this process is helpful to anyone who may be called upon to help with childbirth and to care for the mother and child after the delivery.

Life begins with the union of two different cells: the sperm and the ovum. The sperm cell comes from the male, the ovum from the female. When the sperm cell unites with the ovum through intercourse, fertilization or conception occurs. Growth and development of the fertilized ovum takes place in the female's body and this eventually results in the birth of a child. A study of the female reproductive system will show how it is especially adapted by nature for this purpose.

The female reproductive system has four basic functions:

- To produce ovarian hormones which are responsible for the female sex characteristics and reproductive functions.

- To produce the ovum and deliver it to the place where conception may take place.
- To nurture and sustain the developing fertilized ovum (product of conception) until birth.
- To accomplish delivery of the product of conception.

The external reproductive organs are the external genitals; however, the breasts are also considered to be reproductive organs because they play an important part in pregnancy and lactation. The internal reproductive organs of the female are the vagina, the uterus, the fallopian tubes and the ovaries.

THE EXTERNAL ORGANS

The external genitals are the structures that surround the opening to the vagina. They include the vulva and the perineum. Accessory organs involved in childbirth are the breasts and the anus.

The Vulva

The pad of fat that covers the pubic area is called the mons veneris. It is considered to be a part of the vulva. The vulva consists of two prominent folds or lips called the labia majora, and the structures within them: the labia minora, the clitoris, Bartholin's glands, entrance to the vagina, the urinary meatus, and the perineum.

THE FEMALE REPRODUCTIVE SYSTEM 3

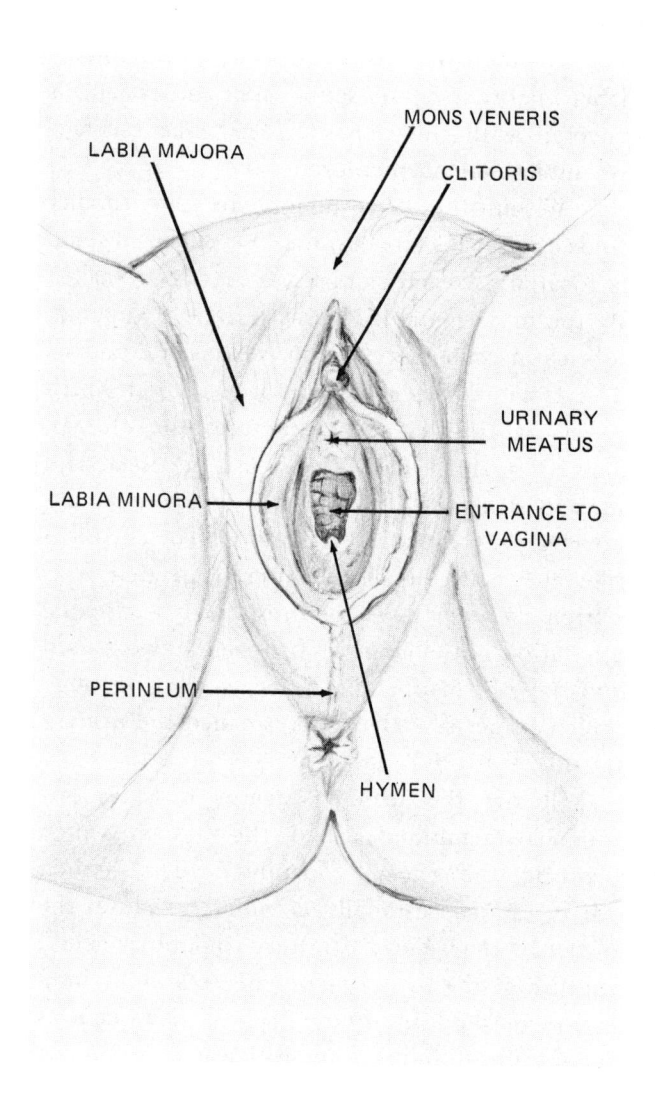

Fig. 1-1 External female genitals

Like the mons veneris, the outside surface of the labia majora is composed of skin and fat and is covered with pubic hair. The inner surface resembles mucous membrane.

Within the labia majora are two smaller folds called the labia minora. A specialized gland is located on each side; these glands are called Bartholin's glands. They secrete a mucoid, lubricating substance during sexual intercourse. The labia minora meet to form a hood which covers a tiny erectile structure, the clitoris. This is a small elongated mass of tissue and muscle richly supplied with blood vessels and covered with mucous membrane. The clitoris is like the male organ, the penis, in that it is extremely sensitive and responds to sexual excitation. Below the clitoris are two raised ridges with an opening between them through which urine is voided; this is called the urinary meatus, figure 1-1, page 3.

Below the urinary meatus is a fold of mucous membrane called the hymen which protects the vaginal opening. The hymen partly (and occasionally completely) closes the outlet of the vagina. Contrary to popular belief, rupture of the hymen is not necessarily an indication of the loss of virginity. It may occur as the result of injury, surgery, use of tampons, active sports, premarital examination, or sexual intercourse.

The Perineum

The area of skin, connective tissue, and muscle which lies between the vagina and the anus, is known as the perineum. The muscle tissues stretch and contract to open and close the vagina and the anus. The perineum stretches to accommodate delivery of the newborn. Injury to the perineum during birth may affect the support of the internal organs and bowel control.

The Breasts

The breasts are considered to be accessory reproductive organs since they play an important part in pregnancy and lactation. They are located over the front part of the chest. As pregnancy progresses, the breasts undergo physiological changes to make ready for the demands of nursing the newborn.

The Anus

The anus lies below the perineum. It is a deeply pigmented, puckered opening which serves as the outlet of the rectum. While not considered part of the reproductive system, the rectum is often used for examining procedures during pregnancy and labor because of its anatomical position. The anus is controlled by a circular muscle called the anal sphincter. This muscle controls the passage of feces and flatus.

6 BEFORE CHILDBIRTH

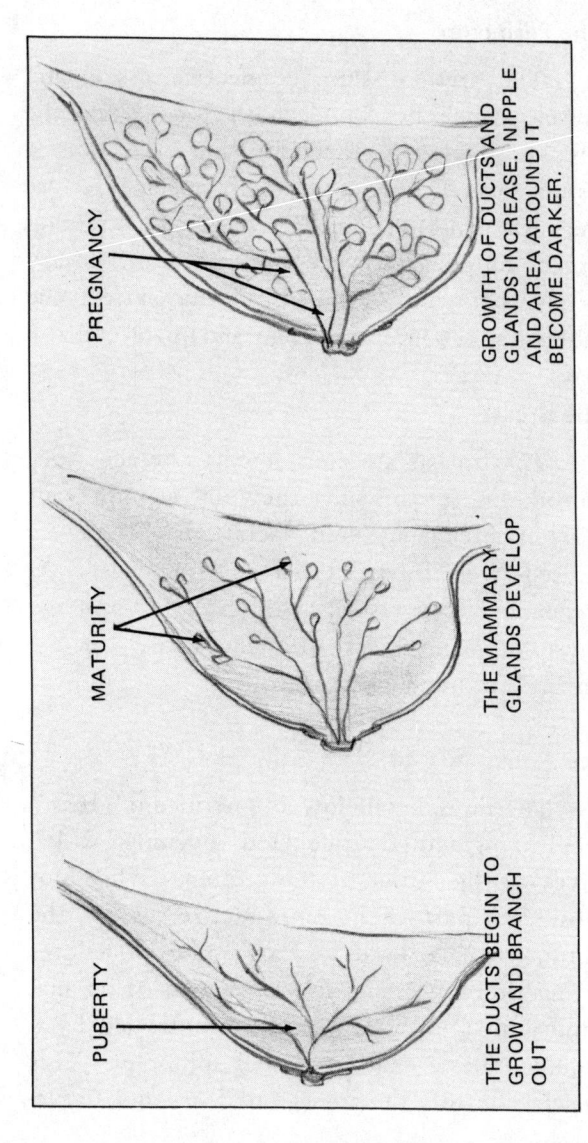

Fig. 1-2 The mammary glands prepare the breasts for nursing the newborn.

THE FEMALE REPRODUCTIVE SYSTEM 7

The mucous membrane of the rectum is very sensitive and easily injured.

INTERNAL ORGANS

The internal reproductive organs are those which lie within the pelvic cavity. They consist of the vagina, uterus, fallopian tubes, and ovaries. Also included are the supporting structures.

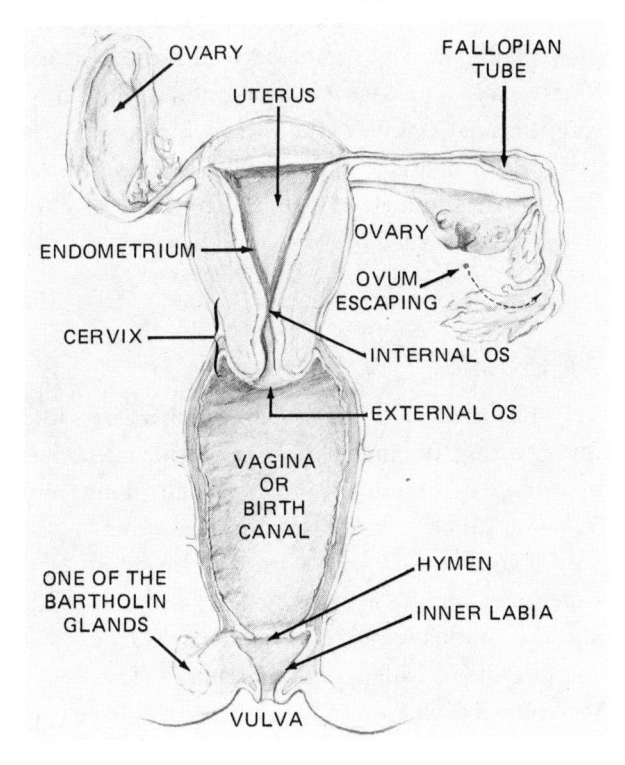

Fig. 1-3 Internal female reproductive organs

The Vagina

The vagina is a tubelike passage leading from the vulva to the uterus. It is capable of great expansion during labor. The vagina is lined with a mucous membrane containing many folds. Located directly in front of the vagina is the urethra and in back of it is the rectum. The secretions in the vagina are largely from the glands of the cervix. The cervix is the lower part of the uterus. The vagina serves four important functions as a passage: introduction of the penis, reception of semen (fluid in which sperm is carried), discharge of menstrual flow and uterine secretions, and delivery of the product of conception. The vagina leads into the cervix of the uterus.

The Uterus

The uterus is the organ which carries the fetus during pregnancy. It is a firm, muscular, pear-shaped organ 2½ to 3 inches long and 3/4-inch thick. It occupies the middle of the pelvis and consists of a narrow lower portion called the cervix (neck), the body (middle part), and the fundus (rounded top part). The lining of the uterus is called endometrium. The endometrium receives and nourishes the fertilized egg.

The cervix of the uterus projects into the vagina. The cervix has a little round passageway called the cervical canal. Uterine secretions, the menstrual flow, the unfertilized ovum, the fetus during labor, and the lochial discharge (vaginal drainage during the six-week period following delivery) pass from the uterus through the cervical canal to the vagina.

The Uterine Ligaments. The broad ligaments are two structures which extend from the side walls of the uterus to the pelvic walls. The ovaries and fallopian tubes are attached to these ligaments. The round ligaments of the uterus, attached to the side walls of the uterus, pass through the broad ligaments to reach the mons veneris. These ligaments help to support the pelvic organs.

The Fallopian Tubes

The two fallopian tubes, or oviducts, extend outward from the upper corners of the uterus to the abdominal cavity. They are about the diameter of a drinking straw and are largely muscular structures. The distal (farthest) portion of each tube curves around and above the ovary in such a way that the fingerlike projections cup over the ovary but are not actually attached to it. Their function is to carry the ovum from the ovary to the uterus. Conception usually takes place in the fallopian tube.

10 BEFORE CHILDBIRTH

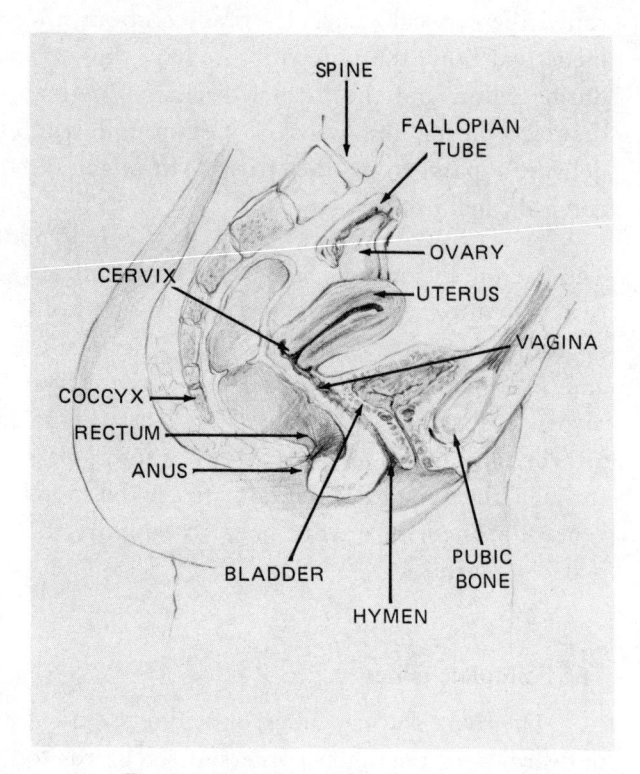

Fig. 1-4 Side view of the female organs

The Ovaries

The two ovaries are also known as the sex glands of the female. In shape and size, each resembles an almond—hard, fibrous, silvery white, and dimpled. After menopause, they atrophy (decrease in size) and shrivel. Their functions are to mature and discharge ova and to produce

THE FEMALE REPRODUCTIVE SYSTEM

hormones necessary to the process of reproduction. At birth, there are several hundred thousand immature ova present in both ovaries. At puberty, the ovaries systematically release a single ovum at a time. This process continues until the time of menopause, unless interrupted by pregnancy or the use of oral contraceptives.

THE PELVIS

A female pelvis can be termed gynecoid (typically womanlike) or android (manlike). The gynecoid pelvis is slightly heart-shaped and is the best shape for childbearing. The android

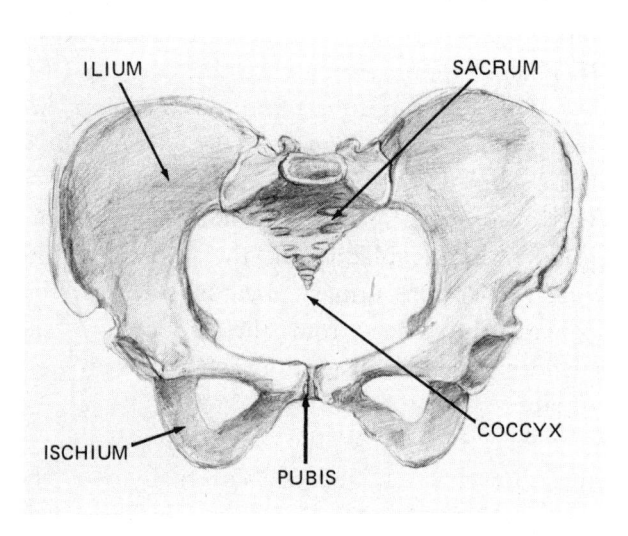

Fig. 1-5 The pelvis is a basin-shaped ring of bone.

pelvis is wedge-shaped and angular and is less suitable for childbearing. The difference between the male and female pelvis is that the male pelvis is heavier, narrower, and deeper.

There are three innominate bones, the ilium, the ischium, and the pubis which form the lateral and anterior boundaries of the pelvis. The posterior wall of the pelvis is formed by the sacrum; it is a large wedge-shaped bone composed of five sacral vertebrae that have fused, see figure 1-5. The coccyx is a small triangular bone made up of four vertebrae fused together and found at the end of the spine. It is connected to the sacrum by a hinge-type joint and forms part of the posterior boundary of the pelvis. The coccyx also helps support the pelvic floor.

Other structures within the pelvis are the bladder, ureters, and urethra. The bladder lies behind the pubis and in front of the uterus. It is a storage space for urine. The urethra leads from the bladder to the opening in the vulva called the urinary meatus. The ureters convey the urine from the kidneys to the bladder. Bladder distention delays the progress of labor.

The rectum is the terminal portion of the bowel. It opens externally to the anus and lies behind the uterus in the pelvic cavity.

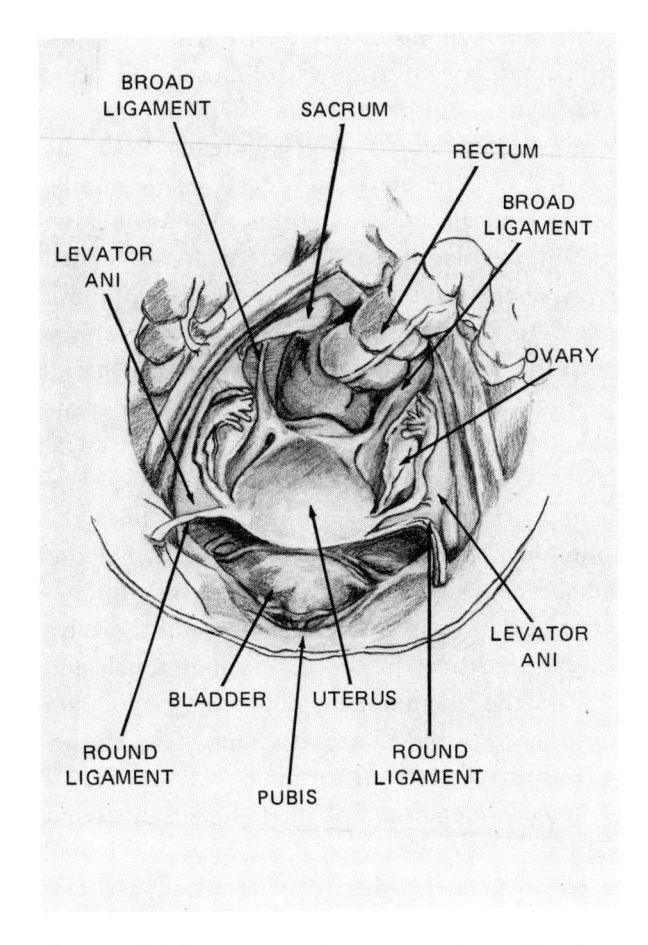

Fig. 1-6 Pelvic structures viewed from above. Note how the underlying levator ani and the other ligaments support the organs of the pelvis.

The Pelvic Floor

The organs in the pelvis are supported by ligaments made up of connective tissue, strands, bands, and layers. A powerful muscle called the levator ani reinforces them. The levator ani forms a "hammock" which extends from the side walls of the pelvis and meets in the middle line around the anus and vagina. The vagina, the rectum, the bladder, and the uterus are suspended by ligaments and fascias above the levator ani.

The internal reproductive organs form a canal for the passage of the ovum and sperm; they contain muscle and connective tissue which is completely lined with mucous membrane. The organs are partly covered by peritoneum, a transparent membrane that lines the abdominal cavity. Characteristics of the mucous membrane vary according to the function required by the part. The membrane of the vulva is very sensitive; in the vagina it is rough and strong; the membrane lining the cervix and uterus is very vascular and strong. The epithelium is a layer of cells forming the surface layer of mucous membrane of the fallopian tubes and uterus. It is covered with microscopic "hairs" or cilia which, by their waving action, assist in transporting the ovum.

-2-
Ovulation and Menstruation

The female reproductive system undergoes great changes during the life cycle of an individual. Even before birth, the reproductive organs are developing and growing. At puberty, however, the reproductive system is mature so that it can function. It is during puberty that the onset of ovulation occurs. During the childbearing years, ovulation and menstruation take place. Reproductive functions diminish at the time of the menopause and gradually cease even though sexual activity may continue.

Puberty

The reproductive organs generally reach maturity during puberty. Puberty is the period of time between the eleventh and sixteenth year of life; it is the period during which the individual becomes capable of reproduction. The size of the external and internal genitals increases. Pubic hair develops. The production of sex hormones is stimulated. These hormones are responsible for development of sex characteristics and the development of the reproductive organs. In the female, the breasts become larger due to the influence of estrogen and progesterone. The production and release of a mature ovum will occur during puberty. Although mammary glands are present in the breasts of both sexes, they normally develop and function only in the female.

THE MENSTRUAL CYCLE

The processes of ovulation and menstruation are interrelated. Ovulation is the process by which a mature ovum is released and the uterus is made ready to receive the fertilized ovum. Menstruation is the process of casting off the unnecessary uterine lining when conception does not occur. The onset of menstruation is often referred to as the menarche.

The pituitary gland is located at the base of the brain. It is made up of two main parts: the anterior lobe and the posterior lobe. The anterior lobe secretes hormones which control the activity of the ovaries. These two hormones are called the follicle-stimulating hormone or FSH, and the luteinizing hormone or LH.

The ovaries contain several hundred thousand microscopic structures called follicles; each follicle is made up of an ovum and cells. These follicles are embedded in the interior connective tissue of the ovary. During the early part of the

OVULATION AND MENSTRUATION 17

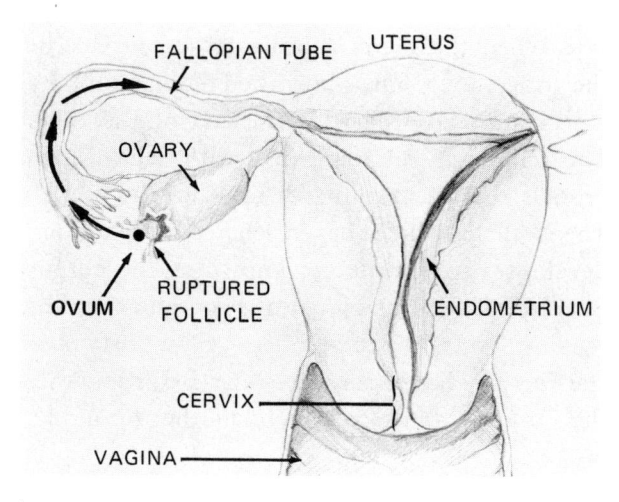

Fig. 2-1 Ovulation: The release of the ovum from the follicle

monthly menstrual cycle, the follicle-stimulating hormone (from the pituitary gland) causes several of the follicles to enlarge and move toward the outside of the ovary. Under the influence of FSH, one of these follicles develops into a small sac in which the ovum develops. This microscopic sac is called a Graafian follicle.

The second pituitary hormone, LH (luteinizing hormone), acts with the FSH in the Graafian follicle to secrete fluid containing estrogen and to cause the developing follicle to rupture after it reaches the outside surface of the ovary. The ovum reaches maturity and is expelled from the follicle. (This takes place about 12-16 days after the beginning of the previous menstrual period.)

When the ovum appears on the surface of the ovary, it is drawn into the fallopian tube by hairlike threads (cilia) at the end of the tube. The fallopian tube is lined with cilia which propels the ovum along its route to the uterus. The follicle which has discharged the ovum, develops into a structure known as the corpus luteum. The corpus luteum is sometimes called "yellow body" because of its yellow fatty substance. The luteinizing hormone (LH) stimulates the corpus luteum to secrete another hormone, progesterone.

Progesterone increases the number and length of the blood vessels in the lining of the uterus and causes secretions. The estrogen (which was in the Graafian follicle before it ruptured) stimulates the glands of the uterine lining to thicken. These changes prepare the uterus to receive the fertilized ovum. At this point, the uterine lining is engorged with blood and is thick and spongy. If conception does not occur, the corpus luteum disintegrates, the secretion of hormones falls off, and a portion of the endometrium (lining of the uterus) is discharged through the vagina. The menstrual flow consists of mucous secretions, tissue fragments, and blood. After menstruation, the endometrium of the uterus is very thin.

If the ovum is fertilized, menstruation does not occur, and the corpus luteum continues to

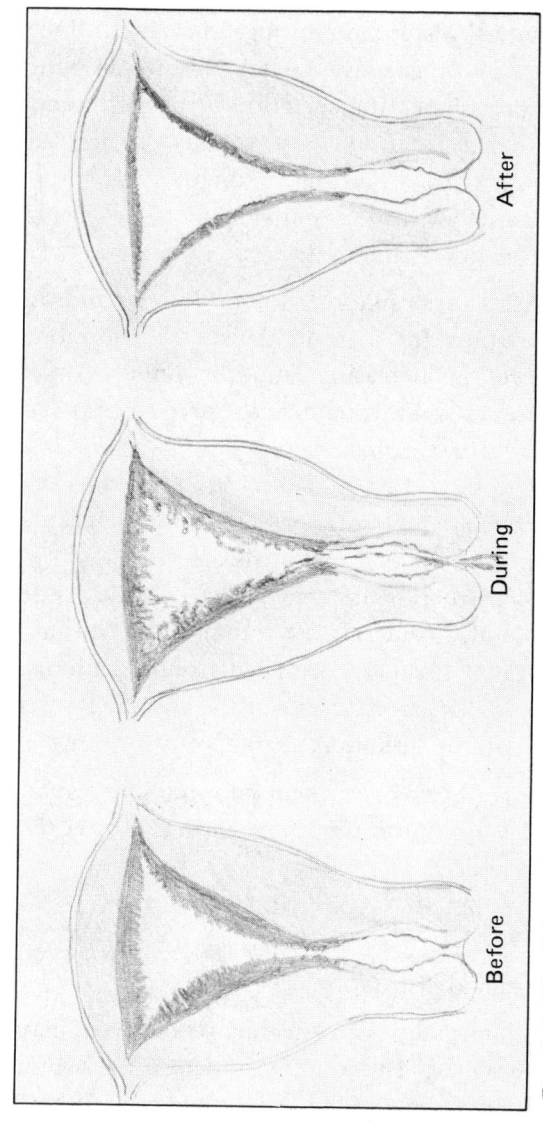

Fig. 2-2 The lining of the uterus changes during the menstrual cycle. Note that it prepares to receive and nourish the ovum during the premenstrual period.

secrete progesterone during the first three months of pregnancy. After this period, the placenta assumes the secretion of progesterone.

A menstrual cycle is usually completed every 28 days. This approximate cycle, however, varies with the individual. The events occurring during the cycle are:

- After menstruation, a period of repair is in progress for 7 to 12 days. The hormone level is increasing, and the lining of the uterus is thickening to prepare for an eventual pregnancy.
- The next 12 to 14 days are known as the premenstrual period. Ovulation occurs around the first day of this period.
- Menstruation lasts from 3 to 7 days while blood, glandular excretions, and disintegrated tissue are expelled from the uterus. The discharge varies but the average flow is about 60 milliliters (2 ounces).

The cycle begins again and continues at regular intervals, except during pregnancy and after the menopause.

Abnormal Menstruation

Abnormalities in the menstrual cycle may be caused by endocrine problems, overwork, change of climate, chronic disease, or other conditions. Some common abnormalities are: amenorrhea, menorrhagia, metrorrhagia, dysmenorrhea, and anovulatory menstruation.

- Amenorrhea — the absence or suppression of menstruation. This may occur as a normal condition before puberty, between menstrual periods, during pregnancy, during lactation, and following menopause. Disease, severe anemia, thyroid imbalance, and psychic upsets can cause amenorrhea. The absence of menstruation may be congenital (existing at birth) or be due to the removal of the uterus. It may also be caused by an obstruction of the cervix or vagina which blocks the external flow.
- Menorrhagia — prolonged or excessive bleeding during the menstrual period.
- Metrorrhagia — bleeding from the uterus at a time other than the menstrual period.
- Dysmenorrhea — painful menstruation. The pain may be due to physical or emotional causes.
- Anovulatory menstruation — menstruation which takes place even though the ovary has failed to expel or discharge the egg. Without ovulation, fertilization of the egg cannot occur. This is one of the causes of sterility in women.

Menopause

Menopause is the permanent physiological cessation of the menstrual flow. The ovaries, uterus, breasts, and external genitalia atrophy. Ovulation ceases, and childbearing is no longer possible.

Menopause, sometimes referred to as the "change of life," is a normal physiological process and is not an illness. Like the menarche, the time menopause occurs varies with the individual; it usually occurs between the ages of 35 and 55.

The tendency to gain weight during menopause is common. Nervous disturbances, hot flashes, and sweating may occur due to the decreased sex hormones and internal secretions. The woman may show signs of anxiety and irritability over a two-to-five year period. Hormone medication may be ordered by the physician to relieve these conditions.

-3-
The Male Reproductive System

The study of childbirth concerns itself with more than the growth of a developing fetus and delivery of a baby. Parenthood includes a mutual sharing of joys and responsibilities. The effects of heredity are as important as the environmental influences. Understanding the father's function and role is also part of the study of childbirth. His support and involvement in fatherhood are important emotionally and physically. This chapter deals with the reproductive process as it involves the internal and external organs of the male reproductive system.

EXTERNAL ORGANS

The external organs of reproduction in the male are the penis and the scrotum. The reproductive cells and secretions are produced by structures within the scrotum and carried to the outside by the penis.

The penis is the male organ of copulation (sexual intercourse). It consists of the urethra and cavernous bodies which resemble a meshwork of spaces. The urethra is used to expel urine or semen. (Semen is the fluid which carries the sperm cells.) The cavernous bodies or blood spaces are usually empty, allowing the penis to be limp. When these spaces fill with blood, the penis becomes enlarged, swollen and erect. The flow of blood is controlled by the nervous system and varies with psychic and physical stimulation. The slightly enlarged structure at the end of the penis contains the opening of the urethra. This part of the penis is called the glans penis. It is enclosed by a fold of skin called the prepuce or foreskin. Part of this skin may be removed for hygienic or religious reasons or because the prepuce is too tight. Removal of the foreskin is called circumcision.

The scrotum is a pouch of loose skin and fatty connective tissue called superficial fascia. Muscle fibers called dartos lie within this superficial fascia. The dartos are subject to temperature conditions. Sperm must be kept approximately six degrees cooler than body temperature or it cannot survive. Heat will cause the dartos to relax, allowing the scrotum to elongate and become limp. This keeps the sperm (which is manufactured by the testes) away from body heat. Cold will cause the dartos to contract, pulling the scrotum upward and closer to the body for warmth. The contracting and relaxing mechanism allows sperm to remain at the most satisfactory temperature. The dartos and the superficial fascia divide the scrotum into two lobes. Each lobe contains a testis and an epididymis. The testis is a small, oblong body; the epididymis is a long coiled tube that rests on and beside the testis. Some other structures are also found in each lobe.

Copulation

Copulation or coitus is the sexual act. Sperm is delivered to the female uterus by insertion of the erect penis into the vagina. Ejaculation is the forcible release of semen from the penis. The amount of semen may vary from 3 to 7 milliliters per ejaculation. (This is about one gram or a little over a teaspoonful.)

Impotent is a term used when a man cannot have an erection or an ejaculation. The cause may be physical, such as a debilitating disease, fever or fatigue, or it may be due to psychological factors such as fear, stress or psychosis (mental derangement). The cure of impotency depends upon the cause. A medical and/or psychological evaluation is often beneficial.

INTERNAL ORGANS

The male's internal reproductive organs are: (1) the testes, which contain the seminiferous tubules, (2) seminal ducts for transporting the sperm from the testes, (3) seminal vesicle glands,

(4) the prostate gland, and (5) the bulbourethral (Cowper's) glands. Semen is a mixture of secretions from the testes, the prostate gland, the seminal vesicles, and the bulbourethral (Cowper's) glands, figure 3-1.

The testes are the primary sex organs of the male; they produce spermatozoa (the mature male sex or germ cell) and the male sex hormone, testosterone. The testes are suspended in the scrotum by spermatic cords and average 4 to 5 centimeters (about 1 1/2 to 2 inches) in length. Each weighs about 10.5 to 14 grams (about 1/2 ounce). Millions of spermatozoa are produced in each testis. Sperm production begins between the ages of nine and fourteen and continues throughout the life of the male.

Each testis is divided into several small lobes that contain tubules. The lining of the tubules consist of sperm-producing cells. These tubules join repeatedly and form the single, coiled tube called the epididymis.

As stated before, the epididymis is a coiled tube, 13 to 20 feet long, located on and beside each testis. It is the principal storehouse for spermatozoa and adds an essential secretion to the fluid in which spermatozoa are activated and stored. This fluid is called semen. Starting in the epididymis, secretions are added as the sperm travels.

THE MALE REPRODUCTIVE SYSTEM 27

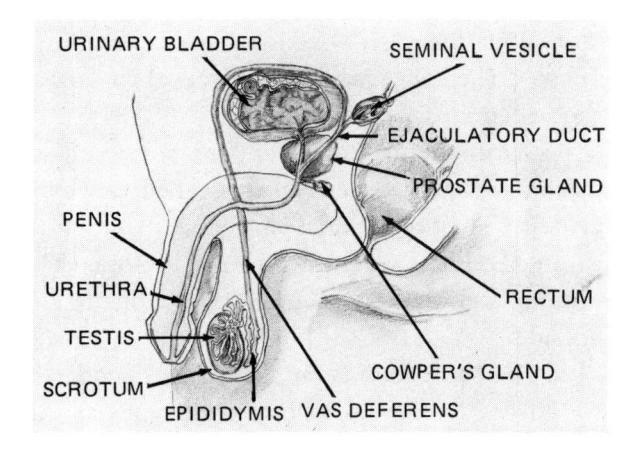

Fig. 3-1 The male reproductive system in relation to the bladder and rectum (side view, vertical section)

From the epididymis, the semen passes through the ductus deferens or vas deferens. The vas deferens is a slim muscular tube approximately 45.7 centimeters in length (18 inches) which carries the semen to the urethra. The urethra serves two purposes in the male — as a passage for semen and as a passage for urine.

Surrounding the urethra at the base of the bladder is the prostate gland, which adds a milky secretion to the semen. This milky fluid is highly alkaline and neutralizes the acidic fluid from the testes in a way that stimulates the sperm to action. Sperm are immobile in acidic media but very active in alkaline media.

Behind the prostate gland are two seminal vesicle glands; they also produce fluid. Their ducts join the vas deferens to form ejaculatory ducts. The two ejaculatory ducts then empty the semen into the urethra.

Below the prostate — on either side of the urethra — are two more glands called Cowper's glands. They also add secretions to the semen through ducts that open into the urethra. The urethra carries the semen and secretions to the outside.

The secretions from the many glands help to lubricate the movement of the penis; this allows the vagina to massage the penis and create the stimulation necessary to release the semen. Without this lubrication, there is an abrasive effect which causes pain, inhibits the sexual desire, and blocks the completion of the sexual act.

Hormone Regulation

Like the ovaries of the female, the testes of a male remain dormant until they are stimulated by the gonadotropic hormones from the pituitary gland. This stage of development is called puberty and occurs between 9 and 14 years of age. The pituitary gland begins to secrete both the follicle-stimulating hormone (FSH) and the luteinizing hormone (LH) which are responsible for the growth and function of the testes. The growth and function of the testes stimulates the release of the primary male sex hormone, testosterone.

Testosterone is derived from cells of the testes and is secreted directly into the bloodstream. Testosterone contributes to:

- Development of the secondary sexual characteristics, such as hair distribution and growth, changes in body contour, and voice changes.
- Sex urge and behavior.
- Development, maintenance, and functioning of the accessory sex organs (seminal ducts, seminal vesicles and prostate gland).

Adolescence extends from puberty to maturity. The reproductive organs of the male continue to function throughout his lifetime. They may, however, diminish in activity as do all body systems as one grows older.

Spermatozoa

The testes of the male produce billions of spermatozoa. Each of these sex cells is made up of a head, a midsection, and a tail. The head is composed chiefly of the nucleus. It carries the genes which are responsible for traits transmitted from the father. The head of the sperm also carries the chromosome which determines the sex of the baby. The tail of the sperm enables the sperm to move about. As long as the sperm

30 BEFORE CHILDBIRTH

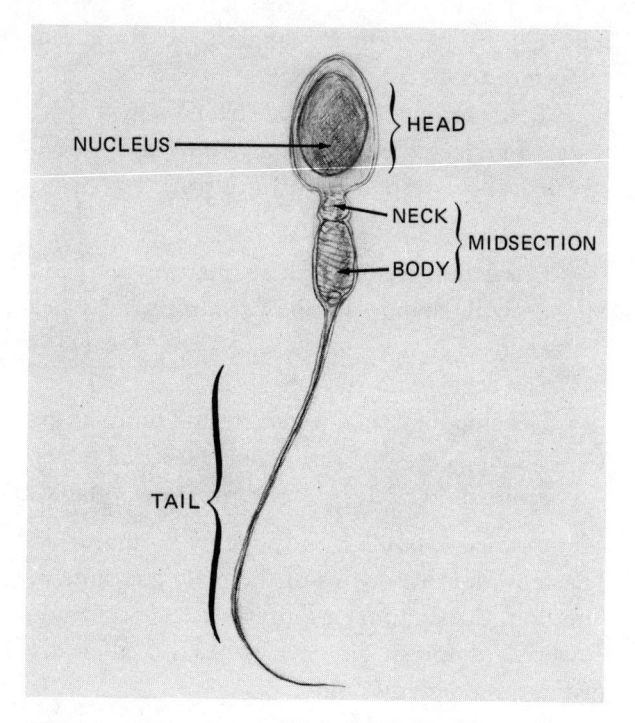

Fig. 3-2 Each sperm consists of a head, midsection, and tail.

remains alive, the tail moves back and forth propelling the sperm forward at a speed of about three inches per hour. This movement allows the sperm to advance into the uterus and up through the fallopian tubes in search of the ovum. Each copulation releases 300 to 1500 million spermatozoa along with secretions from the epididymis, seminal vesicles, prostate and bulbourethral glands. However, only one sperm fertilizes the female ovum. The ovum and the sperm each contribute exactly half of the baby's total hereditary qualities.

STERILITY

About one male out of every 30 is sterile. Sterility may be defined as the lack of viable sperm resulting in the inability to conceive. The most frequent cause of sterility is infection of the genital ducts. A few men have congenitally deficient testes that are incapable of producing normal sperm. Also, undescended testicles may produce sterility. The testes must descend into the scrotum, which is at a cooler temperature, in order to make viable sperm. Undescended testicles produce sterility because the sperm-producing cells cannot live at the warmer, body temperature. Undescended testicles can be corrected surgically, usually before the boy reaches puberty.

Male sterility can also occur when the number of viable sperm falls below 150 million in a single ejaculation. Although it takes only one sperm to fertilize an ovum, it is believed that a large number of sperm are necessary to provide enzymes or other substances that help the single fertilizing sperm reach the ovum. The enzyme known as *hyaluronidase* must be present in sufficient quantity to dissolve the layer of cells surrounding the ovum.

Purposeful sterilization can be accomplished by a relatively simple operation known as a vasectomy. This operation prevents the sperm from traveling beyond the vas deferens. However, it does not interfere with the secretions from the other glands along the seminal pathway. The man who has had a vasectomy can still experience an erection and ejaculation; however, the semen does not contain spermatozoa. A vasectomy is not considered a reversible operation but new surgical techniques are being explored in this area of sterilization.

-4-
The Beginning of Life

During intercourse, sperm are ejaculated from the male penis into the vagina. Microscopic in size, but numbering three to fifteen hundred million, these sperm cells move by means of long thin tails. They quickly wriggle from the vagina to the uterus and then to the fallopian tube in search of the female ovum. In spite of the excessive number of spermatozoa, only one sperm cell fertilizes one egg. Multiple births occur when more than one egg is fertilized or when one fertilized egg divides into more than one embryo (stage of prenatal development between the second and eighth week after conception).

CONCEPTION

The human life cycle begins when the head and neck of the sperm enter the ovum. This usually takes place in the fallopian tubes. The resulting fertilized egg is called a zygote. The zygote is one cell with one nucleus, containing

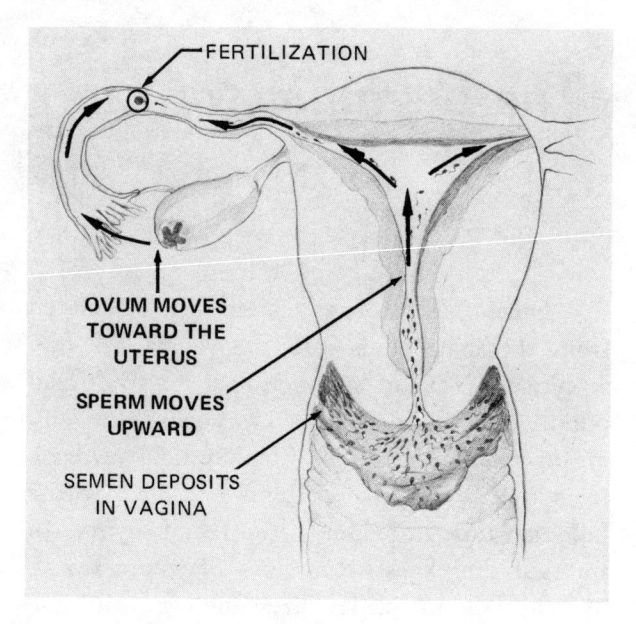

Fig. 4-1 Conception usually occurs in the fallopian tube.

all the necessary elements for the future development of the offspring.

Soon after the nucleus of the sperm has merged with the nucleus of the ovum, a series of cell divisions begins. This process of cell division is called cleavage. It usually starts while the fertilized egg is in the fallopian tube. The egg does not increase in size as the cell division and multiplication continue. It gradually takes on the appearance of a mulberry. The fertilized ovum is traveling down the fallopian tube to the uterus during the cell division. This passage takes seven

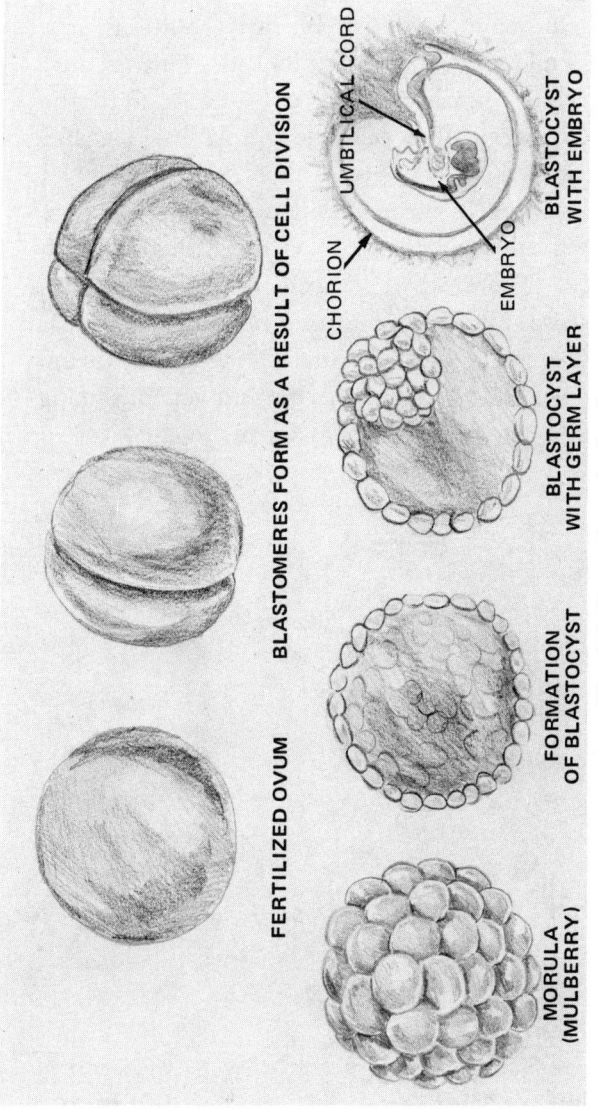

Fig. 4-2 Stages in early development

to nine days. When it reaches the uterus, it is only about the size of a pinhead. This product of conception is called an embryo until the eighth week of development. After the eighth week, it is called a fetus.

The cells meanwhile have regrouped themselves and now form a hollow ball filled with fluid. The disks of the cells near the outer rim develop into the embryo; the outer rim itself forms the fetal membrane. When the ovum reaches the uterus, it digs into the mucous lining of the uterus, which has been prepared for it.

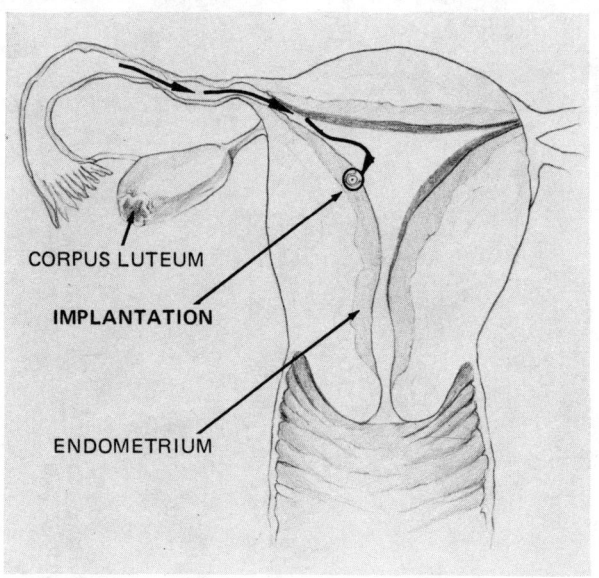

Fig. 4-3 Fertilized ovum attaches to endometrium (lining of the uterus).

DETERMINATION OF SEX

Every cell has a nucleus. The nucleus contains chromosomes; the chromosomes contain genes. Mature sperm cells develop in the testes of the male from the age of puberty. The head of each sperm cell has the nucleus of the cell. It contains 23 chromosomes, one of which is the sex chromosome: X for female or Y for male. The mature ovum also has 23 chromosomes, one of which is the X, or female sex factor.

The fertilized egg resulting from conception contains 46 chromosomes: 23 chromosomes from each parent. One of these is the sex chromosome (sex factor). If the ovum has been fertilized by a sperm cell that carried the X sex factor, the resulting offspring will be female. If the sperm carried the Y sex factor, the offspring will be male. It is the male chromosome that determines the sex of the child. Figure 4-4, page 38, describes this in more detail.

HOW TRAITS ARE INHERITED

Geneticists study heredity and its variations. These scientists have established that certain traits are transmitted through the genes. Genes determine hereditary traits and are found in the chromosomes. The chromosomes are made up of chains of giant molecules, a combination of protein and nucleic acid.

38 BEFORE CHILDBIRTH

22 chromosomes and 1 sex chromosome (X) from ovum
plus
22 chromosomes and 1 sex chromosome (X) from sperm
} 44 + 2 X chromosomes = female child

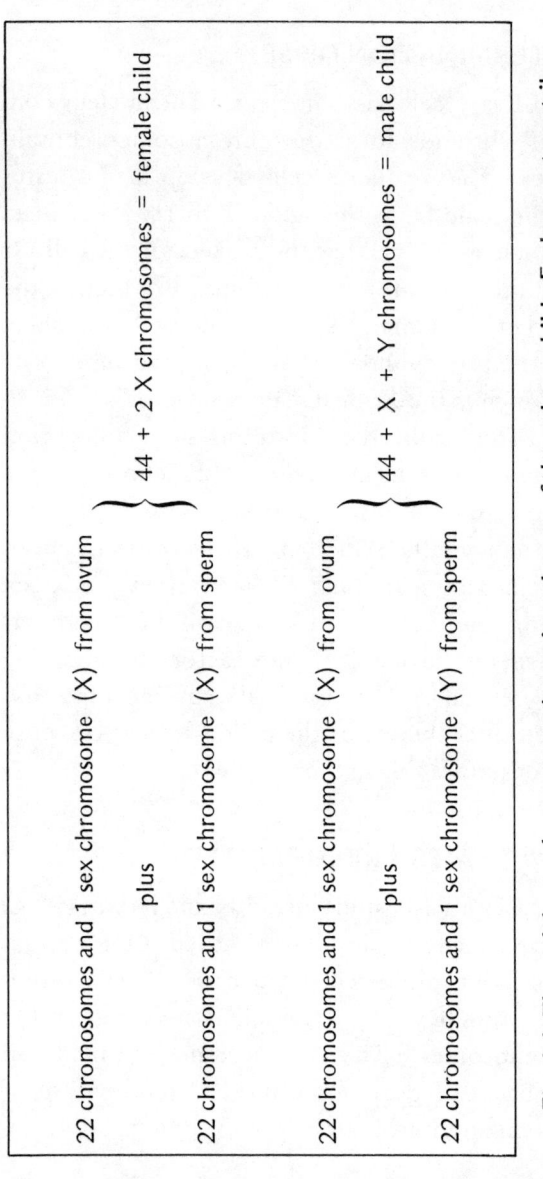

22 chromosomes and 1 sex chromosome (X) from ovum
plus
22 chromosomes and 1 sex chromosome (Y) from sperm
} 44 + X + Y chromosomes = male child

Fig. 4-4 The male's sex chromosome determines the sex of the unborn child. Each parent contributes 23 chromosomes, one of which has the sex factor.

The nucleic acid in the chromosomes is called DNA or deoxyribonucleic acid. DNA contains the full genetic information needed for the formation of the human body; it could be called the master template for cell building. Histones are also present in the chromosomes. Histones are a class of simple proteins derived from the nucleus of cells. It is believed that histones have a major function in all cell differentiation. This means that the histones block out part of the DNA information and leave open only that information needed for the cell to become a certain kind of cell such as a liver cell, bone cell, etc. Another nucleic acid, present outside the chromosomes, is RNA (ribonucleic acid) which is involved in protein building.

It is known that some physical traits are associated with the genes in the X and Y (sex) chromosomes. These are referred to as sex-linked characteristics. Color blindness is a sex-linked characteristic. The trait is believed to be linked to the female (X) chromosome. Therefore, it can be transmitted from grandfather to grandson through the grandfather's daughter. Hemophilia, a disease in which the blood fails to clot, is also a sex-linked characteristic. If a male hemophiliac produces a daughter, she would carry one normal X chromosome (from her mother) and one hemophiliac X chromosome (from her father). She would not be a hemophiliac since the healthy X chromosome would mask the hemophiliac chromosome. If, however, she had a son, he could receive either a normal or a hemophiliac X chromosome from his mother. If he received a hemophiliac chromosome from the mother, he would have the disorder since he has no healthy X chromosome to mask the hemophiliac chromosome. A female would be a hemophiliac only if she inherited a hemophiliac chromosome from both her parents.

Sex-limited characteristics are traits that appear in one sex only. It is believed that traits for the development of beards and baldness in men belong to this category.

In addition to sex-limited characteristics, traits are said to be dominant or recessive. The dominant trait requires only a single gene and is more likely to appear since it can mask another trait. A recessive trait will appear only when a pair of like genes is present. Some dominant traits include dark hair, brown eyes, farsightedness, astigmatism, curly hair, glaucoma, cataract, and susceptibility to rupture. Among the recessive traits are blue or gray eyes, nearsightedness, light hair, Rh-negative blood type, diabetes mellitus, and congenital deafness. Sometimes, characteristics may be due to two recessive traits rather than to the dominant one.

MULTIPLE BIRTHS

Twins are described according to their origin. Identical twins result from the union of one sperm cell and one ovum. Fraternal twins result when two ova are fertilized by two sperm cells. In identical twins, the fertilized egg divides into two embryos. There is one placenta and two amniotic sacs; the twins

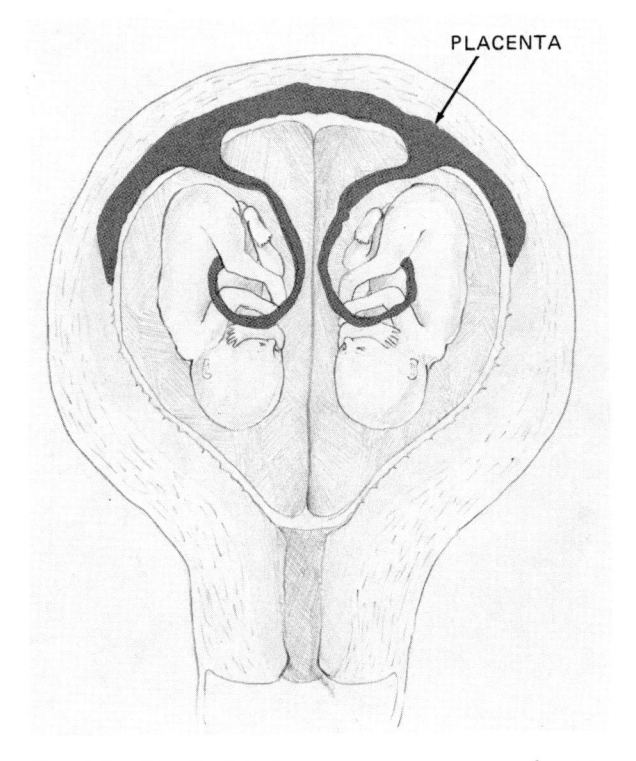

Fig. 4-5 Identical twins: two sacs — one placenta

are always the same sex. Fraternal twins may or may not be of the same sex. They have two amniotic sacs and separate (or fused) placentas. Heredity has been recognized as a factor in the production of identical twins. Age of the mother seems to be a factor in the production of fraternal twins; in older women, more than one ovum may be released during ovulation.

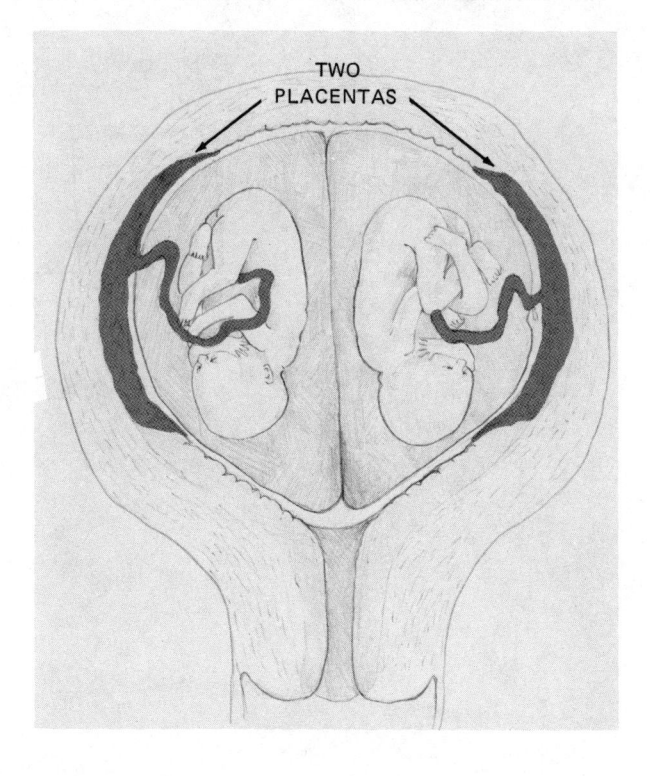

Fig. 4-6 Fraternal twins: two sacs — two placentas

-5-
Prenatal Development

During the first to second week after conception, the fertilized ovum forms a blastocyst while it travels down the fallopian tube, enters the uterus, and becomes implanted in its lining. Once firmly implanted in the endometrium (uterine lining), the rapid growth of the embryo begins. The embryo develops from the second to the eighth week after fertilization. Then it becomes a fetus and continues to develop until the time of birth. Prenatal development may be divided into three trimesters; this division of time makes it easier to understand what takes place — and when — from the time the ovum has been fertilized until the fetus is ready to be born. The average length of pregnancy is about 9 calendar months or 10 lunar months. A lunar month is 28 days.

DEVELOPMENT OF THE EMBRYO

The first 28 days following conception is the first lunar month. By the end of the first

44 BEFORE CHILDBIRTH

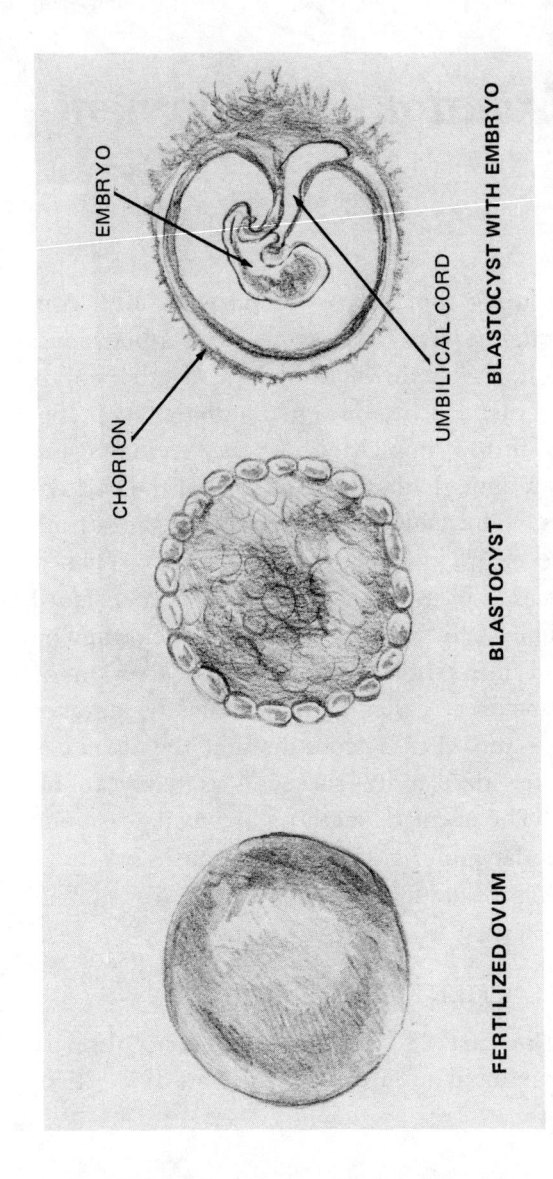

Fig. 5-1 The embryo develops from the fertilized ovum which, through cell division, has developed into a blastocyst.

lunar month, traces of all organs become differentiated and rudiments of the eyes, ears, nose, and limbs appear. Development of the embryo proceeds from head to tail.

During the next 28 days, or second lunar month, the head becomes larger because the brain is developing. Facial features are relatively small. The external genitals appear but cannot be clearly identified although the sex has already been determined at conception. The embryo is about one inch long. The circulatory system is established between the mother and the embryo through the umbilical cord. The cord is attached to the mother's uterine wall and to the embryo's navel, in the middle of its abdomen. The average length of the umbilical cord is about 20 inches although the length may vary from 7 inches to 4 feet. The cord contains 2 arteries, which take waste products from the developing fetus to the placenta to be excreted by the mother, and one vein, which carries nourishment and oxygen to the embryo and developing fetus.

The Amniotic Sac

A fluid-filled sac develops around the embryo. This sac is formed by the amnion which is a smooth, transparent inner fetal membrane. The amnion grows rapidly and by the end of the eighth week it fuses with the outer fetal membrane called the chorion. The fusion of the amnion and the chorion forms the amniotic sac which is more commonly known as the "bag of waters."

The embryo is suspended in the amniotic sac by amniotic fluid. Amniotic fluid is slightly alkaline, transparent and almost colorless. It equalizes the pressure around the fetus and keeps it moist. The fetus floats and moves about in the fluid; this keeps the fetus at an even temperature and cushions it from injury. The amount of fluid increases as the fetus develops. At the time of birth, it varies from 500 to 1000 milliliters (one pint to one quart of fluid).

DEVELOPMENT OF THE FETUS

Centers for bone formation are laid down in the long bones during the third lunar month. The fingers and toes can be distinguished. The nails begin to form, and the external genitals show some sex distinction. The fetus resembles a human form, weighs about 15 grams (1/2 ounce) and is now 9 centimeters (about 3 1/2 inches) in length.

If the fetus is expelled from the uterus at this time, it will not survive; this is a miscarriage or an early spontaneous abortion. A large number of miscarriages which occur in the early months of pregnancy are believed to be caused by imperfect implantation or embryonic formation.

At the beginning of the second trimester of pregnancy, the fetus looks like a baby with the eyes closed. The arms and legs are short; the fingers and toes, well-formed. Fingernails are beginning to grow, and the teeth are developing in the gums. During the second trimester (4th through the 6th month) downy hair called lanugo begins to appear on the shoulders and back. The skin is wrinkled.

The fetal heartbeat can be heard as early as the thirteenth week with a sensitive instrument called the fetone. By the twentieth week, the fetal heartbeat can be heard with a fetoscope. It is about this time that the mother-to-be notices movement of the fetus. This movement is known as quickening.

By the end of the fifth lunar month the fetus weighs about 10 ounces and measures 10 to 13 inches in length. Should it be born at this time, it will be extremely frail. Its expulsion from the uterus could be called a late abortion. Most states require a fetal death certificate if the fetus is expelled at this time. If the fetus shows any signs of life, a birth certificate is issued.

During the third trimester (7th to 10th lunar month) the fetus becomes covered with a cheese-like substance called vernix caseosa which acts as a protection to the skin. Since the fetus is surrounded by fluid, a softening of the skin could occur if there were no protective coating.

Deposits of fat begin to form under the very thin skin of the fetus. The bowel contains a thick, dark green substance called meconium. This is made from bile, mucus, and cells. Meconium will be the newborn's first bowel movement.

The eighth lunar month can be called the month of storage. It is at this time that the supplies of iron, calcium, phosphorus, and nitrogen — needed for continuing development and immediate use after birth — are being stored. The fetus is now fully developed and weighs nearly three pounds. If there should be a premature termination of pregnancy, the fetus would be able to survive. However, special care is necessary if it is to live.

In the ninth and tenth lunar months, the fetus gains weight rapidly, about 8 ounces per week, because of the subcutaneous (under the skin) fat deposits. The hair and nails are fairly long. The fetus begins to shed the downy hair (lanugo) and may even suck the thumb. The fetus born at nine lunar months has an excellent chance of survival.

1st Lunar Month
Length 7.5-10 mm (0.1-0.16 inches)
Eyes, ears and nose begin to appear.
First traces of all organs become differentiated.
(Remember: A lunar month is 28 days — just less than a calendar month.)

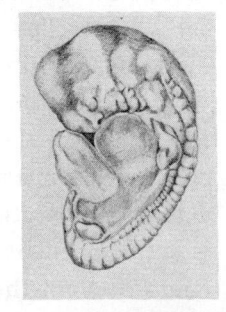

2nd Lunar Month
Length 2.5 cm (1 inch)
Embryo markedly bent.
Extremities begin to show.
Head very large, because of development of brain.
External genitalia appear but sex cannot be determined.

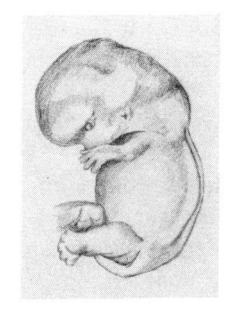

3rd Lunar Month
Length 7-9 cm (2.8-3.6 inches)
Fingers and toes distinct, with soft nails.

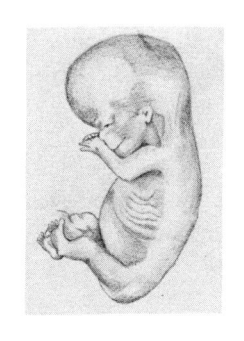

4th Lunar Month
Length 10-17 cm (3.9-6.7 inches)
Weight 55-120 gm (1.9-4.2 ounces)
Sex can be definitely differentiated.
Downy hair (lanugo) appears on head.

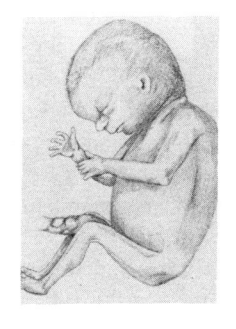

5th Lunar Month

Length 18-27 cm (7.1-10.6 inches)
Weight 280-300 gm (9.9-10.6 ounces)
Lanugo over entire body with small amount on head.
Fetal movements usually felt by mother.
Heart sounds can be perceived.

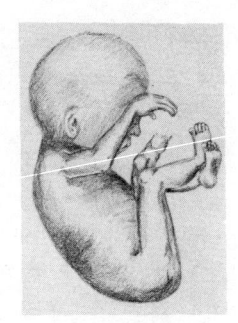

6th Lunar Month

Length 28-34 cm (11.1-13.4 inches)
Weight 650 gm (1.4 pounds)
Skin wrinkles.
Eyebrows and eyelashes appear.
If born, fetus does not survive.

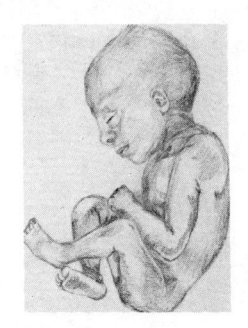

7th Lunar Month

Length 35-38 cm (13.8-15.0 inches)
Weight 1200 gm (2.6 pounds)
Skin red and covered with vernix.
Pupillary membranes disappear from eyes.
If born, fetus breathes, cries, moves but usually dies.

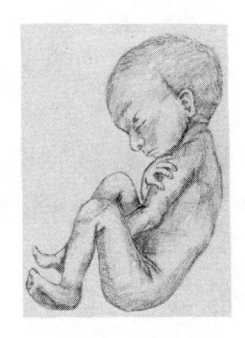

PRENATAL DEVELOPMENT 51

8th Lunar Month
Length 38-43 cm (15.0-17.0 inches)
Weight 1600-1900 gm (3.4-4.2 pounds)
Appearance of "little old man."
If born, may live with proper care.

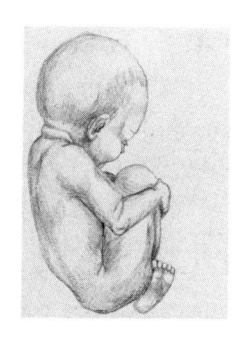

9th Lunar Month
Length 42-48 cm (16.6-18.9 inches)
Weight 1700-2600 gm (3.7-5.7 pounds)
Face loses wrinkled appearance due to subcutaneous fat deposit.
If born, good chance to survive.

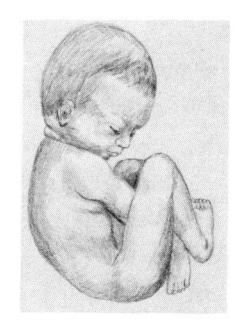

10th Lunar Month
Length 48-52 cm (18.9-20.5 inches)
Weight 3000-3600 gm (6.6-7.9 pounds)
Skin smooth, without lanugo (except about shoulders), covered with vernix.
Scalp hair usually dark.
Fingers and toes with well-developed nails projecting beyond their tips. Eyes uniformly slate colored; impossible to predict final hue.

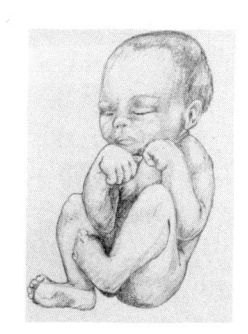

PRENATAL CARE

Certain factors may influence the development of the embryo. The pregnant woman who follows a well-balanced diet feels better and is more apt to retain her health than one who chooses her food thoughtlessly. Quality rather than quantity is the main consideration. Studies have shown a relationship between the mother's diet and the health (and size) of the baby at birth. Activity, rest, and recreation are necessary.

Pregnant women tire easily. Fatigue must be avoided. Normal activities in recreation and housework may be continued but should not be excessive. A woman who does her own housework needs little additional exercise. However, she does need fresh air, sunshine, and diversion. Walking is valuable, both for the maintenance of correct carriage and posture and for its value in getting the patient into the fresh air. Any activity which incurs sudden jolts, changes of momentum, or physical trauma should be avoided. Sports may be enjoyed at a mild pace. Adequate rest periods should be planned.

If a woman is employed, she should stop working six to eight weeks prior to the expected date of confinement. However, there are cases where, *under the doctor's advisement*, a woman may work longer if she feels well.

The doctor should be contacted when a menstrual period is 2 to 4 weeks late (between the 6th to 8th week of pregnancy). In this way the estimated date will be more accurate. While under the doctor's care, a pelvic examination can be made to determine the size and shape of the uterus as well as the capacity of the pelvic bones. If there is any question about the capacity of the pelvic bones, the doctor will consider ordering an X ray during or prior to labor. X rays should never be taken during early pregnancy.

Usually a complete physical examination is done and laboratory tests are ordered. Prevention and treatment of infectious diseases and other medical conditions will help the expectant mother and the developing fetus. Diet and weight control are discussed. If the mother's diet is deficient in protein, vitamins and minerals during pregnancy, the child's future mental and physical development may be retarded. If the mother has diabetes, there is an increased possibility of spontaneous abortion, stillbirth, and congenital defects. Babies born to diabetic mothers are usually larger than normal; too much amniotic fluid, causing overdistention of the uterus, is also common. In addition to meeting the physical needs, the doctor and expectant parents form a relationship that meets emotional needs as well.

Frequently the expectant mother is unaware of the pregnancy. She may take drugs which are harmful to the developing embryo and result in malformations. Thalidomide is an example of such a drug but there are others.

The pregnant woman may contract infectious diseases. German measles (rubella) may cause cataracts, mental retardation, deafness, and abnormalities of the heart in the developing embryo. In order to prevent deformities in the developing embryo, it is suggested that young girls be given the rubella vaccine before their reproductive years.

Syphilis is another infectious condition that may affect the development of the embryo. The requirement for a Wasserman or other blood tests before marriage has reduced the incidence of deformities due to venereal disease. However, some unmarried couples become parents and the unborn child may be infected. If the fetus should be infected before the fifth month, it will probably die. If syphilis was contracted by the mother in the later months of pregnancy and inadequately treated, the baby will be born with congenital syphilis. This condition affects the heart, long bones, skin, and respiratory system of the fetus; it may cause premature delivery or the birth of a stillborn (dead) infant.

Scarlet fever and smallpox are two other infectious diseases contracted by the mother-to-be that may interfere with normal embryonic development. Immediate treatment of streptococcal sore throats and proper immunization reduces the possibility of harm to the embryo.

Serious problems arise if the nourishment of the mother or the oxygen level of her blood is deficient. The common cold, heavy smoking, pneumonia, extreme anemia, and heart failure are dangerous since they interfere with the circulation of adequately oxygenated blood to the placenta. If the brain of the fetus does not receive sufficient oxygen (from the placenta by way of the cord), brain damage may result.

Another factor which may adversely affect the fetus is a multiple pregnancy. Because of intrauterine crowding, premature birth may result. One of the fetuses may not receive enough minerals and vitamins. Therefore, it is less developed and smaller than the other fetus. Sometimes one survives at the cost of the life of the other.

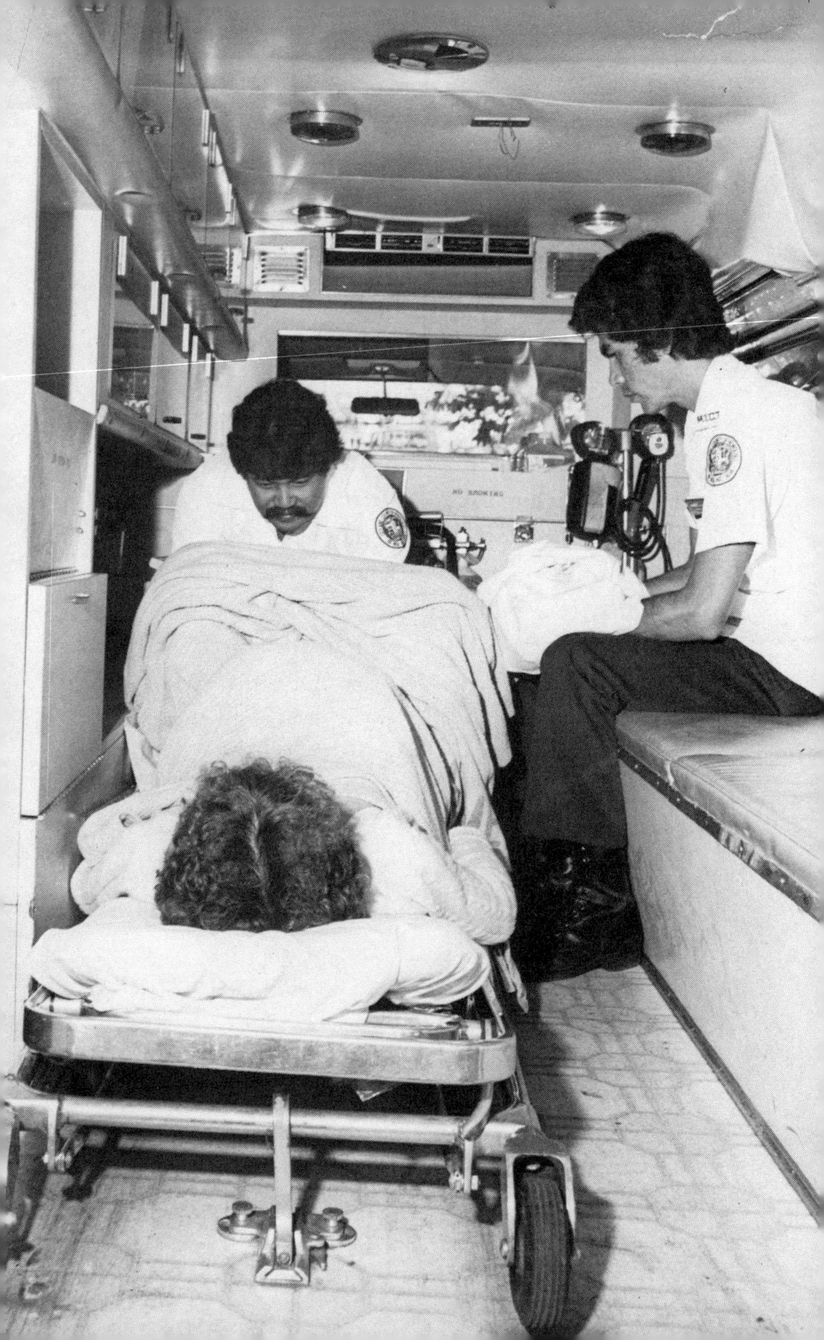

SECTION 2
LABOR AND DELIVERY

-6-
Understanding Labor

Labor is the process by which the baby, the placenta, and the amniotic sac and fluid are expelled from the mother's body. The word labor itself signifies hard work. During labor there are many physical sensations within the mother's body that occur at no other time. Feelings of anticipation, excitement, satisfaction, fear, pain, disbelief, disappointment, happiness, sadness, and relief may all be experienced during the period of pregnancy to parenthood.

Labor is an involuntary process. It usually begins at just the right time — when the fetus is mature enough to cope with conditions outside the uterus. The average woman who is having her first baby is called a primipara. She may spend about 15 hours in labor. The woman who has had a child is called a multipara. She may spend 10 hours or less in labor. The times are extremely variable. Generally a range from 3 to 24 hours is considered to be within normal limits.

What causes labor to begin is not fully understood. Each labor is unique, differing from labor to labor for the same woman and from one woman to another. However, certain changes do take place to prepare the uterus for delivery of the baby. During the early weeks of pregnancy, uterine contractions called Braxton-Hicks contractions begin and continue periodically throughout gestation. They are painless and the woman is usually not conscious of them. These contractions enlarge the uterus in order to accommodate the growing fetus; they also develop the uterine muscles needed to expel the baby. They become more noticeable toward the end of the pregnancy and may sometimes be erroneously taken for labor pains.

In the final two to four weeks, the fetus drops into the pelvis; this effect is called lightening. The fundus of the uterus lowers, making

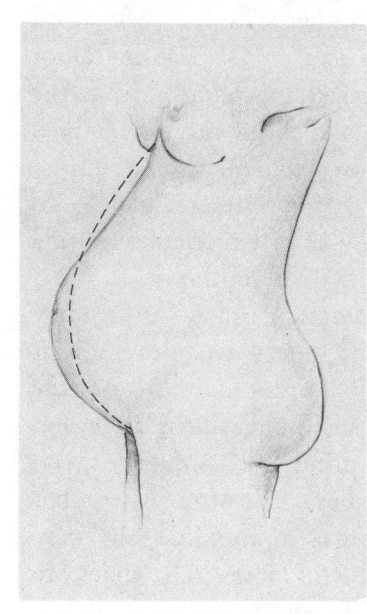

Fig. 6-1 Lightening takes place shortly before the first stage of labor. The fetus drops into the pelvis (called the engagement position).

the upper part of the abdomen flatter and lowering the waistline. Breathing becomes easier, but walking and moving about are more difficult. As in early pregnancy, the pressure of the uterus causes frequency of urination.

SIGNS OF LABOR

One or more signs may indicate that labor has begun: (1) a vaginal discharge called the "show", (2) regular contractions, or (3) rupture of the bag of waters. Frequent reference will be made to these signs throughout the text, so it is best to understand them at this time.

The "show" is a vaginal discharge consisting of thick, stringy mucus streaked with blood; this is caused by the rupture of small blood vessels in the cervix and lower segment of the uterus. (Before discharge, it was a mucous plug located at the opening of the uterus — the cervix.) If there is actual bleeding at any time, it is considered abnormal and the doctor must be notified.

Regular contractions of the uterus are intermittent; that is, there are periods of relaxation between them. The early contractions are usually short and mild, lasting 30 to 40 seconds. There are 3 parts of each labor pain: the contraction begins and increases in intensity; the contraction is at its highest; and then the intensity of the contraction decreases. In other words, every contraction has a buildup, peak, and decline. The most severe pain is felt at the peak of the contraction.

A period of relaxation follows each contraction before another one starts. This period between contractions is called an interval. At the beginning of labor, the intervals may be as long as 20 minutes. Labor pains may be described, for example, as lasting 40 seconds and being 20 minutes apart. As labor progresses, the intervals become shorter. Generally speaking, a woman with labor pains which are two minutes apart is close to delivery.

Rupture of the bag of waters is the tearing of the membranes containing the amniotic fluid which supported the baby during the pregnancy. The amniotic fluid is a colorless, water-type liquid. It may gush or trickle out of the vagina, depending on the degree of tear in the amniotic sac. Sometimes the bag of waters will not break until after the labor pains or contractions have begun. Other times it may break before contractions start.

Some signs that indicate labor is not progressing normally are:

- Abnormal vaginal bleeding.
- Contractions stop after labor has begun.
- A rise in blood pressure.
- A rigid uterus after contraction has stopped.
- Severe headache and dizziness.

- Passage of meconium-stained fluid (unless baby is in breech position)
- Umbilical cord is seen at the vaginal opening (prolapse)

There are many questions about labor. What makes the contractions start? What happens during a contraction? What causes the pain? There are several theories. One of the most widely accepted theories concerns the action of a hormone produced by the posterior lobe of the pituitary gland. This hormone is called *oxytocin*. For some unknown reason, when the baby is ready to be born, the gland secretes more oxytocin than it normally does. The oxytocin is discharged into the blood, where it is carried to the uterus. Oxytocin causes contractions of the uterus.

During a contraction, the uterus hardens and rises. This exerts a pull on the cervix. (The cervix is the lower narrow portion of the uterus.) The ligaments that support the uterus are also pulled during the contraction. Oxygen supply is reduced in the contracted tissue. The cervix continues to stretch and dilate. All of these factors contribute to the pain of labor. In addition, the pressure of the baby's head against the cervix stimulates the release of more oxytocin, so further contractions take place. The uterine contractions and cervical dilation continue until the cervix has dilated to about 4 inches (10 centimeters). This is enough to allow the baby to descend into the vagina to be born. After childbirth, the oxytocin helps contract the uterus and return it to its normal, pre-pregnant size.

THE STAGES OF LABOR

Labor proceeds in 3 stages. The first stage extends from the time the cervix (opening to the uterus) begins to widen until it is complete. This is called the period of dilatation. The second stage is the period between complete dilatation of the cervix to the delivery. This is called the period of expulsion. The third stage begins with the birth of the child and lasts until the afterbirth (placenta) is expelled. The last stage is known as the placental stage.

Stage 1: Period of Dilatation

Although labor varies in length, the first stage is about 15 hours long for the woman who is bearing her first child. It is sometimes difficult to determine exactly when labor begins because contractions may start before dilatation of the cervix starts. Dilatation may be slow or rapid depending upon the age of the patient, her general physical condition, and the number of previous pregnancies.

The woman has begun the first stage of labor when:

- Regular contractions become stronger and last longer while the intervals between them are shorter.
- The mucous plug that forms in the cervix during pregnancy is discharged. This is usually tinged with blood and is known as the "show."
- Changes take place in the cervix; these are identified by a rectal or vaginal examination, performed by a doctor or other qualified experienced practitioner.

Sometimes the bag of waters may rupture before the mother-to-be goes into labor. Breaking of the bag of waters can happen suddenly, followed by a gush of fluid, or it may be noticed as a slow, uncontrollable leaking of fluid. If the bag of waters ruptures, the woman should be brought to the hospital immediately. Infection or other complications (such as prolapse of the baby's cord) could take place. It is important to note the exact time the membranes rupture because it helps to determine the time of delivery. Also the color of the fluid and the amount (estimated usually as teaspoonfuls) should be reported.

The entire first stage of labor is involuntary; nothing can be done except to help the mother relax. NEVER urge her to push or bear down during this stage. Forceful pushing when the cervix is not completely dilated can make it puffy and swollen. This can make the opening smaller because of the swelling, thereby delaying delivery. In addition, the mother's strength diminishes and she will not be able to help at the time of the birth because of exhaustion.

The labor pains become more intense as the cervix dilates. By the time the woman has reached the last phase — when the dilated cervix is about 3 inches — she may be very tired. This last phase is sometimes referred to as the transition phase. It is the shortest but the most difficult time of all. The woman has very little rest between contractions; her uterus is working very hard. She may become restless, withdrawn, and appear unaware of her surroundings. Burping, nausea, and vomiting may occur. She may feel very warm and perspire freely. Her face is flushed, she is very uncomfortable, her legs may tremble, and she may have a backache. She may feel the pressure of the baby in her pelvis; this can be compared to the urge to have a bowel movement. The intensity of the activity within her body may almost overwhelm her. Although every woman will not experience all of these discomforts, every pregnant woman will usually experience some of them at this stage. She needs assistance and as much emotional support as possible. The presence of someone who understands and

CERVIX CLOSED
AND THICK
BEFORE LABOR
BEGINS

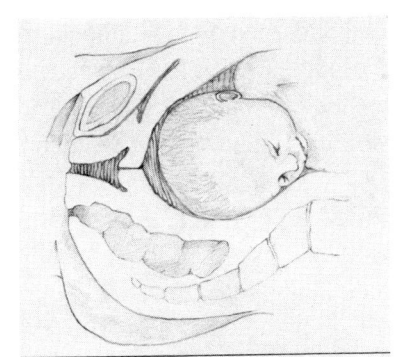

CERVIX BEGIN-
NING TO DILATE.
NOTE HOW THIN
IT HAS BECOME.

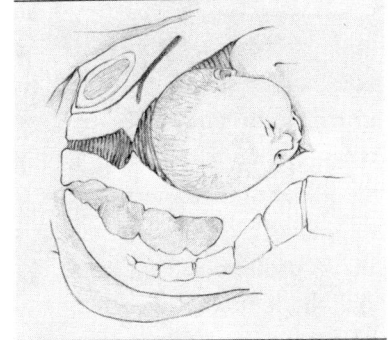

CERVIX FULLY
DILATED: THE
END OF THE FIRST
STAGE OF LABOR.

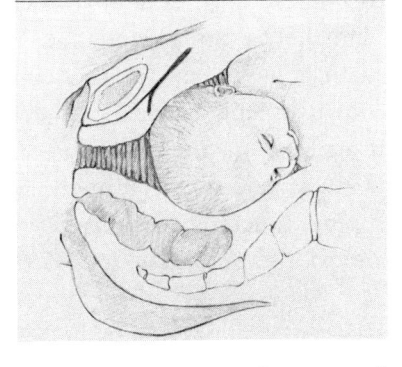

Fig. 6-2 Changes in the cervix during the first stage of labor (dilatation).

is concerned is very important. Sometimes the husband is with her during this trying period and he can help her. If he is not available, others should encourage the woman and help her.

Stage 2: Period of Expulsion

The second stage of labor begins after the cervix is fully dilated (4 inches or 10 centimeters). Usually a short period follows, without contractions. When they resume, the mother is able to play a more active role in this second stage of labor. During the first stage, there was nothing she could do to hasten or help with the delivery. In the second stage, she may be encouraged to take a deep breath, hold it, and bear down with each contraction so that the abdominal muscles contract and help to expel the baby. As the contractions lengthen in duration and become more frequent, the vaginal tissue bulges and the rectum stretches. More and more of the baby's head can be seen as it gradually moves down the birth canal. The mother's perineum bulges from the pressure of the baby's head. Finally the head crowns as it stretches the vaginal opening. A burning sensation called the "rim of fire" may be felt by the mother.

The most painful moment of this second stage of labor is when the fetal head passes over the stretched perineum. At this time, the mother should not push, but allow the baby's head to slowly glide out of the vagina. As the head emerges, it slides over the perineum usually face down. It then turns 90° to face the mother's thigh, figure 6-3, page 70. The shoulders emerge followed by a gush of water and blood and the wet, slippery body.

Stage 3: Placental Stage

After the baby has been born, it is still connected to the mother by the cord. The umbilical cord is attached to the placenta (in the mother's uterus) and the baby's navel (belly button). The contractions continue for a time before the placenta separates. These contractions are not severe at first; they become stronger to expel the placenta. The placenta is squeezed by the contractions and falls away from the uterine lining. (Bleeding from the vagina occurs at the time of separation of the placenta.) When completely separated from the uterine wall, the placenta slides down into the lower part of the uterus. In order to expel it, the mother may push with the contractions as she did when delivering the baby. **Caution**: NEVER pull on the cord to hasten delivery of the placenta. Severe hemorrhage could result.

After the placenta has been expelled, the uterus contracts. The uterus becomes hard and

70 LABOR AND DELIVERY

A. Crowning

B. Head passes over the perineum

C. Head is born

D. Head turns 90° to face mother's thigh

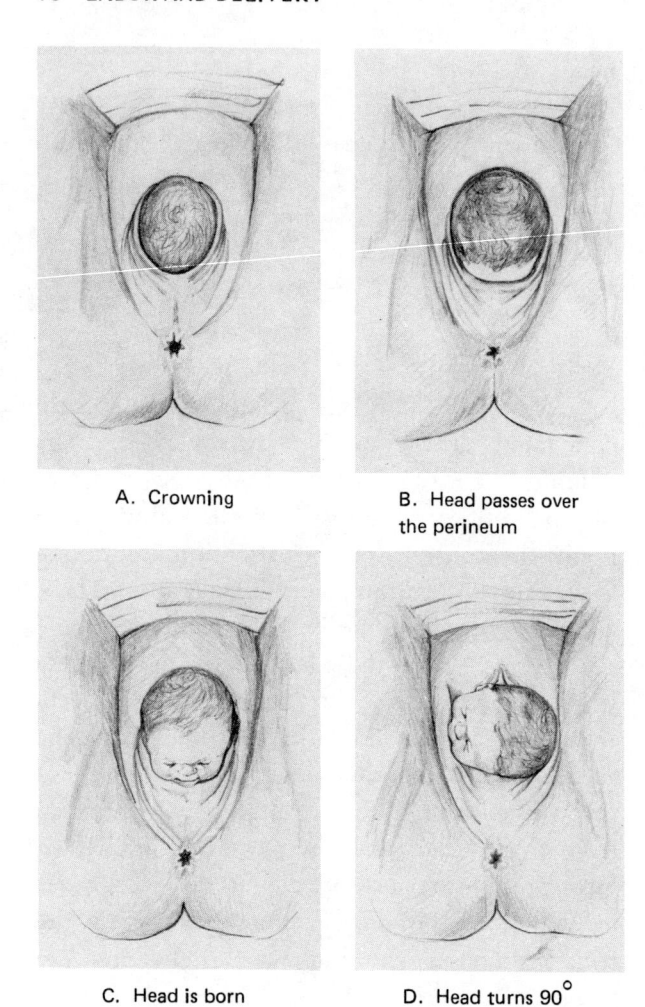

Fig. 6-3 Progress of the baby as it emerges during the second stage of labor (Continued)

UNDERSTANDING LABOR 71

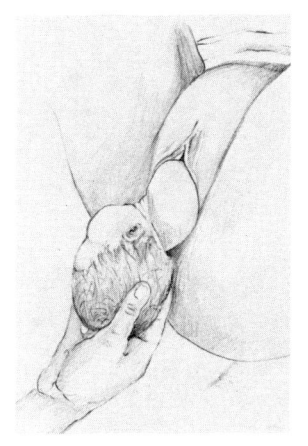

E. Upper shoulder delivers

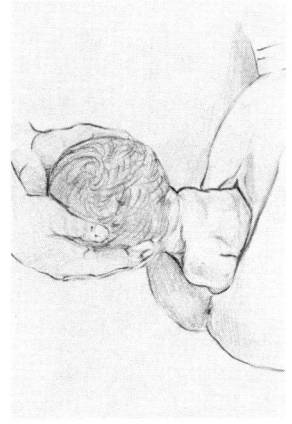

F. Lower shoulder delivers

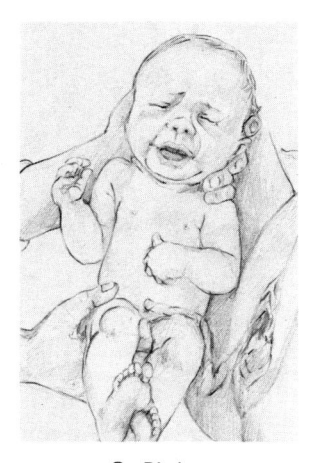

G. Birth

Fig. 6-3 Progress of the baby as it emerges during the second stage of labor (expulsion)

72 LABOR AND DELIVERY

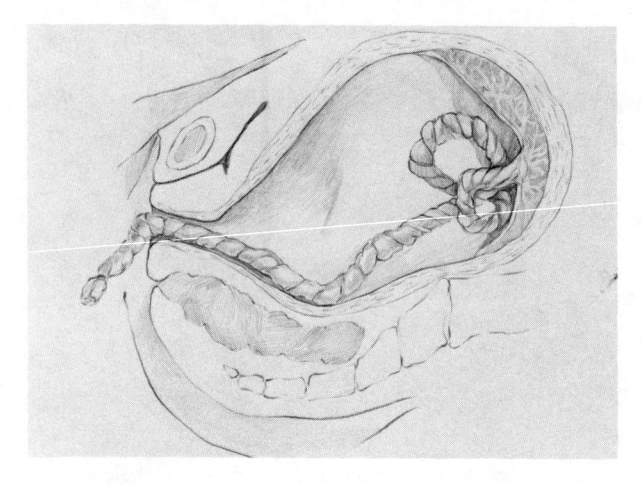

A. Contractions squeeze the placenta making it fall away from the lining of the uterus.

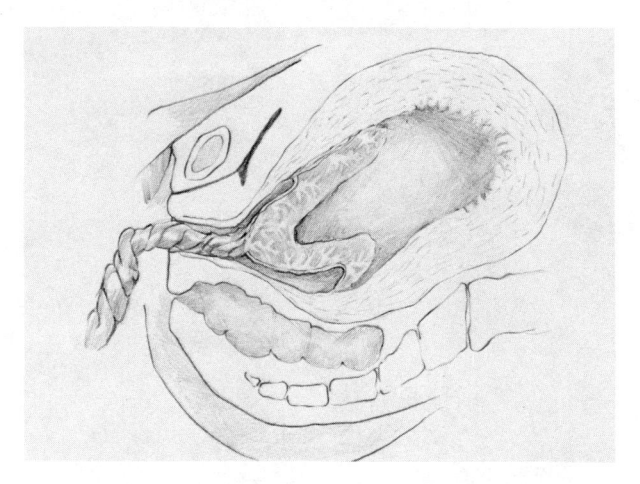

B. The placenta slides down into the lower part of the uterus and is expelled by the mother's pushing with the contractions.

Fig. 6-4 The third stage of labor (placental)

firm and once more lies in the pelvis where it was before pregnancy. The fundus (top part of the uterus) can be felt through the mother's abdomen, just below her navel. If the uterus rises or becomes soft, this could be a symptom of hemorrhage. It is most important that it be carefully massaged until it becomes firm and remains so.

FALSE LABOR

It is often hard to tell if a woman is in labor. Sometimes contractions may occur a few days to a few weeks before labor actually begins. These abdominal cramps may be due to gas in the bowel or to the normal irregular contractions which were described before (Braxton-Hicks sign) and which may occur throughout a normal pregnancy. These pains are annoying and may resemble true labor. However, false labor differs from true labor because false labor contractions are:

- usually confined to the lower abdomen
- irregular in frequency, intensity, and duration
- not always painful
- usually longer, from 3-4 minutes
- relieved by a warm bath or slight activity such as walking

On the other hand, true labor has contractions which usually radiate from the back to the front of the abdomen; they are regular and gradually increase in frequency, intensity, and duration; contractions are accompanied by a tightening feeling in the abdomen, pain or discomfort; they seldom last over one minute; and they are not relieved by any activity — even mild medication fails to relieve these contractions.

Examination of the cervix, done by the doctor or other medically qualified practitioner, reveals no change if the woman is experiencing false or pre-labor contractions. In the case of true labor, the cervix would show signs of shortening and dilating, and the mucous plug (show) would be present in the opening to the cervix.

MECHANISM OF LABOR

It is important to know the relationships of the baby and the birth canal in order to understand the mechanism of labor. The terms, *presentation* and *position* are used to describe these relationships.

Presentation refers to the relation of the long axis of the baby to that of the mother. In most cases, this axis is parallel to or in the same plane as the mother's and is called a longitudinal presentation. A much rarer occurrence is a transverse presentation in which the baby lies across the mother's pelvis. The presenting part

UNDERSTANDING LABOR 75

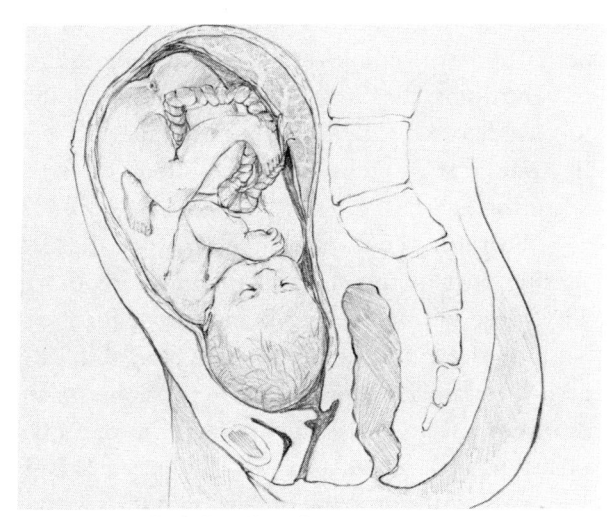

LONGITUDINAL PRESENTATION

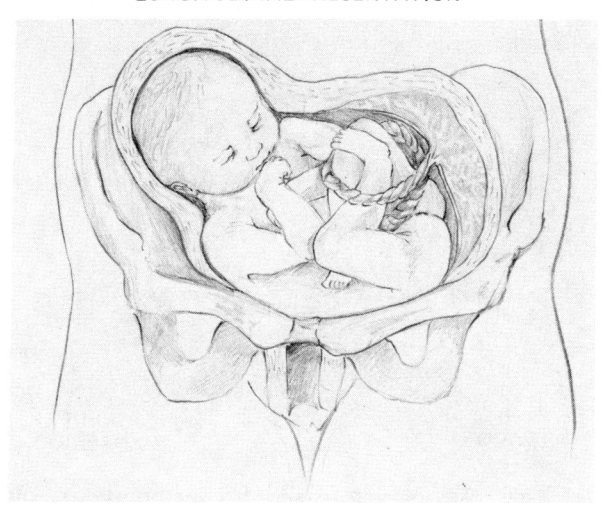

TRANSVERSE PRESENTATION

Fig. 6-5 Two presentations: longitudinal and transverse

76 LABOR AND DELIVERY

is the part of the fetus which is lowest in the pelvis and will come out first. In longitudinal presentations the presenting part may be either the head, the buttocks, or occasionally the feet. In transverse presentations the shoulder is the presenting part.

Position refers to the relation of the presenting part of the child to the mother's pelvis. The space within the pelvic inlet is divided into four sections to show the right and left sides and the anterior and posterior portions of the mother's pelvis. If the baby is in the LOA position, this means its head (occiput) is in the left, anterior part of the mother's pelvis. The left occiput anterior (LOA) position is the

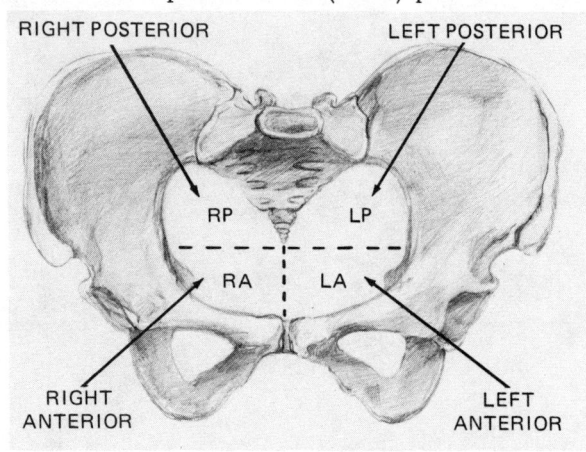

Fig. 6-6 To understand and describe position of the fetus, it is necessary to divide the pelvic inlet into 4 sections: anterior and posterior, right and left.

UNDERSTANDING LABOR 77

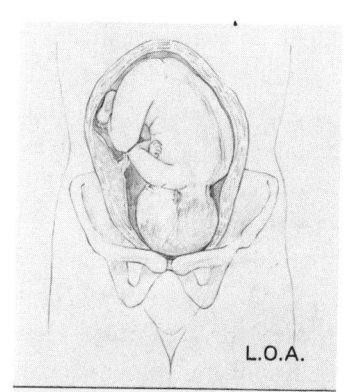

Fig. 6-7 Three positions: Note the relation of the presenting part to the mother's pelvis (*O* refers to occiput or head, *S* refers to sacrum or end of spine). *A* refers to anterior part of mother's pelvis and *L* and *R* refer to left and right side.

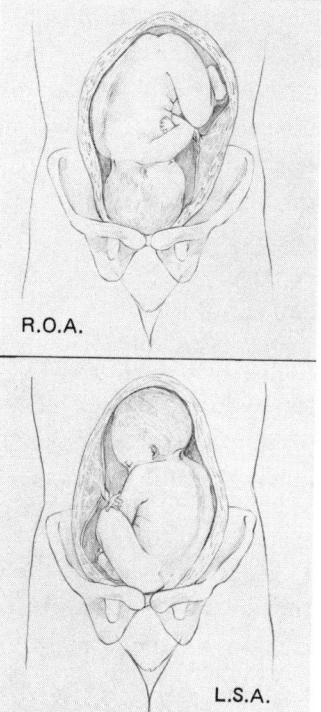

L.O.A.

R.O.A.

L.S.A.

most common position and the most favorable for the welfare of the mother and baby.

If the baby is in ROA, this means the head is on the right side of the anterior part of the mother's pelvis. If the baby is in the LSA position, the sacrum (buttocks) is on the left side of the anterior part of the mother's pelvis.

The position of the fetus must change as it passes through the pelvis and birth canal. A series of movements, called the mechanism of labor, adjusts the position so that the smallest possible area of the presenting part encounters the irregular shape of the pelvic outlet. In this way, the fetus will meet as little resistance as possible as it passes from the mother's body. In order of occurrence, the movements are engagement, descent, and flexion; followed by internal rotation, extension, external rotation, and expulsion.

Engagement. Engagement is the shift of position which takes place during lightening — the presenting part descends and fully enters the pelvis. In multiparas, engagement sometimes does not occur until labor begins.

Descent. Descent is the continuous progress of the fetus as it passes through the birth canal. It is brought about by the downward pressure of uterine contractions. Descent begins after the presenting part of the fetus has entered the pelvis; that is, when engagement is accomplished. More and more of the baby's head can be seen as it gradually moves down the birth canal. The mother's perineum bulges from the pressure of the baby's head.

Flexion. As the fetus descends and the head encounters resistance, flexion occurs. The head of the fetus is bent forward so that the chin rests on the breastbone. Flexion is important because the narrowest part of the head must enter the pelvic outlet.

Internal Rotation. Internal rotation takes place mainly during the second stage of labor. When engagement takes place, the baby's head enters the pelvic inlet in a tranverse or diagonal position. In order for the baby's head to emerge from the pelvic outlet, it turns its head 45 to 90 degrees to the left. This turning is called *internal* rotation because it takes place within the uterus. If the fetus must move from a posterior position (as in the case of an LOP), it may have to rotate as much as 135 degrees. This means a longer labor with much more discomfort for the patient.

Extension. When the head of the fetus passes out of the pelvis and is stopped under the pubic arch, it cannot make further progress unless extension occurs. At this time the head becomes unflexed and pushes upward out of the vaginal

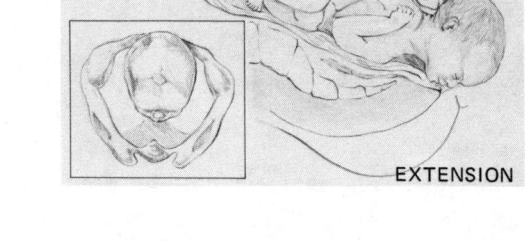

Fig. 6-8 Mechanism of labor showing positions of the fetus as it adjusts to the irregular shape of the pelvis.

EXTERNAL ROTATION

EXPULSION

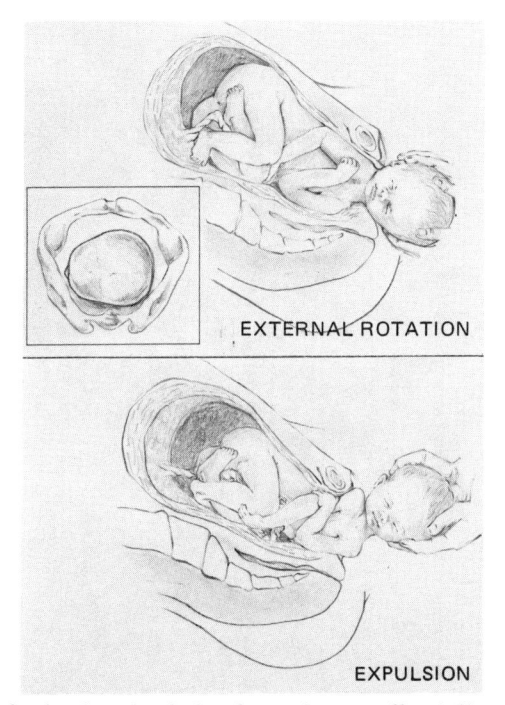

canal; the head of the fetus is actually delivered during extension. As the head crowns, the nape of baby's neck pivots on the lower surface of the mother's pubic arch and the face slides over the perineum.

External Rotation. After the head is delivered, it rotates back 45 to 90 degrees or until it resumes its normal relationship with the shoulders. The rotating of the head during external rotation helps to line up the unborn shoulders.

Expulsion. The final movement in the mechanism of labor is the delivery of the shoulders and body.

RELIEVING DISCOMFORT DURING LABOR AND DELIVERY

First Stage — DILATATION	From beginning of contractions to complete dilatation of the cervix.
Contractions —	Encourage the woman to relax during contractions and to breathe deeply through her mouth.
Backache —	Apply pressure to the small of the back. Rub her back briskly. Have her turn from side to side after every few contractions.
Perspiration —	Sponge face and hands with cool water.
Anxiety —	Reassure the woman in a calm, confident manner. Keep her informed as to what is happening.
Fatigue —	Encourage her to relax. Help her assume positions of relaxation such as lying on her side with one knee and thigh drawn up, or the tailor-sitting position.
	Tell the woman not to bear down at this stage of labor.
Full bladder —	Encourage her to urinate whenever she feels it is necessary.
Irritability —	Understand that a woman may be irritable at this time and accept it cheerfully.

RELIEVING DISCOMFORT DURING LABOR AND DELIVERY

Second Stage — EXPULSION	From complete dilatation of the cervix to expulsion of the baby.
Urge to push —	Ask the woman to bear down with each contraction.
Fear of having a bowel movement —	Assure her that this is a normal sensation and there is no need for embarrassment.
Leg cramps —	Stretch the leg out and pull foot toward the knee. If this does not relieve the cramp, apply warm towel to the leg.
Dry lips —	Apply cold cream or baby oil to the lips.
Anxiety —	Explain what you are going to do before you do it. Keep her informed as to what is happening. Encourage and reassure her in a calm, confident manner.
Sweating —	Sponge face and hands with cool water.
Crowning —	As the baby's head emerges, tell the woman not to push. She can relax by taking quick short breaths, puffing her cheeks, and blowing the air out with each breath.

Third Stage — PLACENTAL	From expulsion of the baby to delivery of the placenta.
Soft uterus —	Massage the top part of the uterus (through the lower abdomen) until it becomes firm.
Profuse bleeding —	Massage uterus until firm; cross the woman's legs tightly; elevate the lower half of her body; encourage the baby to nurse; seek medical help immediately.

-7-
Emergency Delivery

When an untrained person encounters a woman in labor, usually the first thought is to get the woman to the hospital as quickly as possible. If the hospital is some distance away, the baby may be born on the way; sometimes under unfavorable conditions. Therefore — before any action is taken — the state of the woman in labor should be evaluated to see how far labor has progressed. This is necessary in order to estimate how much time is available before delivery can be expected. If birth is likely to occur within a few minutes, it is better to immediately prepare for the birth at the present location. If you do not know the woman, introduce yourself by stating your name. Ask the woman her name. Tell her you can help but you will need her cooperation. In order to evaluate the progress of labor, you will need to know:

1. if this is her first baby
2. how long she has been in labor
3. length of time between contractions

(Temporary notes may be written on page 204 of this book.)

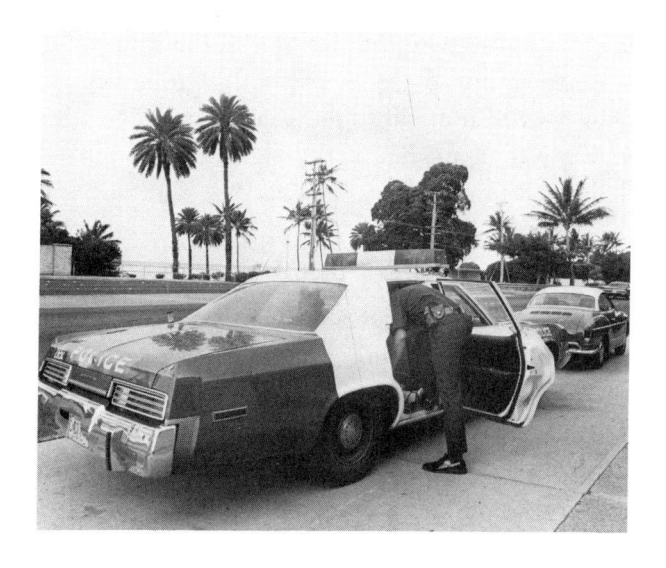

It may become necessary to transfer the expectant mother to the larger police car if there is no time to reach the hospital.

A woman having her first baby usually is in labor for about 12 to 15 hours. If the woman has not been in labor long, there probably is enough time to get her to a doctor or hospital. However, it is not unusual for the labor to last from 3 to 24 hours. If this is not the first baby, she may have a much shorter period of labor. Keep in mind that the period of time for labor varies considerably; even the woman in labor with her first baby may have a very rapid course of labor. If the time from the beginning of one contraction to the beginning of the next contraction is two minutes or less, the woman is close to or already in the second stage of labor; delivery will normally take place quite soon. It is important to know the signs that indicate delivery is imminent.

SIGNS OF IMMINENT DELIVERY

Knowing the signs that indicate birth will take place within a short time is important when deciding whether or not the woman has time to be taken to the hospital. If the woman is experiencing any of the following, prepare for delivery:

- The interval — time between contractions — is 2 minutes or less.
- The woman is straining or pushing down with the contractions.
- The woman feels she must move her bowels.
- The woman is crying out warning the baby is coming.
- The baby's head can be seen at the vaginal opening at the time of contractions.

In order to determine if the baby's head can be seen, the vaginal opening must be examined during a contraction. Explain to the woman why this examination is necessary. It is important to ask her permission to perform the examination. Avoid embarrassing her as much as possible. If the baby's head can be seen, there will not be much time, so *quickly prepare for delivery*. **Caution**: Never hold the woman's legs together or attempt to delay the delivery in any way. Death could result to both the woman and the baby if this is done.

PREPARING FOR THE DELIVERY

1. **Provide Privacy.** If the birth is occurring in a public place, shield the scene from the view of others. If there are no mechanical barriers to provide the privacy, ask others to form a circle around the woman, with their backs to the delivery scene.
2. **Explain.** Tell the mother-to-be what you are going to do before you do it. This will relieve anxiety and promote relaxation.
3. **Position.** Help the woman to lie on a firm surface, with her knees bent and legs spread apart. Be sure her head is elevated. A pillow or pile of clothing may be used. **Caution**: If she is flat on her back, the baby's weight on the large blood vessel that runs up along the right side of her spine can block the blood returning to the heart. This, in turn, could block the flow of blood to the uterus, cutting off oxygen supply to the baby.

   Place clean towels or folded linen under the buttocks. Newspaper or clothing can be used if nothing else is available. If the birth should occur at home, a plastic sheet may be used to prevent staining the mattress and bed linens. A side-lying position may be used for delivery if the woman is feeling dizzy and unable to stay in the semi-reclining position. For example, if she feels dizzy, or there is a drop in the fetal heart beat, or if the baby is in the ROP or LOP position. Occiput-posterior positioned babies can cause severe back pain which would make side-lying a more comfortable position for delivery.

4. **Drape.** The woman should remove clothing from the lower half of her body. Four clean towels (or sheets) are necessary for draping. One is placed directly under the buttocks, another is placed on the lower abdomen, each thigh is also covered with a towel or sheet. When properly draped, only the vaginal opening is exposed. If towels or sheets are not available, newspapers or clothing can be used for draping. Draping provides a sanitary environment for the newborn and also saves unnecessary embarrassment.

5. **Scrub.** Thoroughly scrub your hands and arms with soap and water up to the elbows. Wash under running water and use much friction; give special attention to the finger-

nails. If it is available, apply an antiseptic such as alcohol to the hands and arms and allow it to dry. If sterile gloves are available, they should be put on after the scrubbing procedure is completed.

6. **Comfort.** Encourage the woman to relax as much as possible and to let her uterus do the work. Encourage her to relax and breathe deeply through her mouth during the contractions. Speak to her in a calm, confident manner. If a basin or pan is available, place it near her head. She may

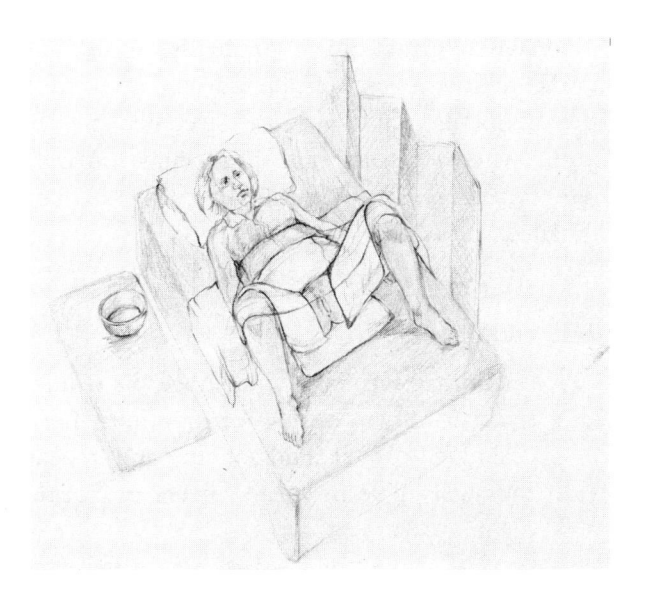

Fig. 7-1 Position and drape for delivery. Provide privacy. Note placement of 4 towels or sheets.

be nauseated and perhaps vomit; especially, if she has eaten recently. It is important that she does not run the risk of choking on the vomited material.

DELIVERING THE BABY

After the scrub, observe the progress of the presenting part as the baby moves forward toward the outer world. Since the presenting part is usually the head, part of the baby's scalp will first be seen. It has a cheesy appearance. At first it will be visible only at the height of each contraction. Gradually more and more of the baby's head will be seen until the perineum and anus are stretched to the point where the hair and head bulge outward due to the pressure of the baby's head. This is called "crowning."

THE HEAD IS SEEN

1. **Encourage Pushing.** Encourage the woman to bear down during contractions for a period of 10 seconds, hold, and repeat. This will move the head further out of the vagina.
2. **Prevent Infection.** Do not touch the perineum or the baby. Infection must be prevented. Due to the bearing down

by the mother, contents of the lower bowel might be expelled at this time. If so, remove the fecal contents and keep the area clean. If necessary, wipe any remaining feces away from the rectum with a downward motion (toward the mother's back). **Caution:** Do NOT wipe toward the vaginal opening. Infection to the child and mother could occur. If your hands should touch the feces, scrub them over again with soap and water — thoroughly.

3. **Reassure and Inform.** Encourage the mother and remind her to keep her thighs and pelvic floor relaxed as much as possible between contractions. Keep her informed of her progress. This is a difficult stage and the most exhausting, painful time of labor. Encourage pushing *until the head is about to emerge*.

4. **Discourage Pushing. Promote Breathing.** As crowning progresses and the head is about to emerge, ask the woman to stop pushing. Tell her that taking short breaths of air, puffing out the cheeks, and then blowing out the air through pursed lips will help her relax. Panting can also be done. Breathing exercises help to deliver the head more slowly and so lessen the risk of tearing the delicate tissues of the mother's perineum.

THE HEAD EMERGES

5. **Guide and Support.** Guide and support the head as it emerges. Place one hand below the vaginal opening to keep the baby away from contact with the mother's rectal area. Use the other hand to support the baby's head as it is delivered. **Caution:** Do not allow the baby to pop out. Do not pull the baby. The purpose is to guide it out of the vagina.

   Spread your fingers evenly around the baby's head while supporting it. This is extremely important as the baby's skull is very soft and finger pressure into the soft area could easily damage the brain. Spreading the fingers distributes the pressure while giving more support at the same time.

6. **Help Baby Breathe.** The baby's head emerges face down. After it is born, the head will turn sideways to face the mother's thigh. Now, the main purpose is to help the baby breathe:

   - Remove Mucus and Fluids. Once the head has fully emerged, use a clean cloth to wipe away any mucus from around the baby's nose and mouth. **Caution:** Do not wipe inside the mouth. You may block the passage of air into the baby's lungs.

     If the membranes are still intact and the head is surrounded by what looks like a cellophane bag, use your fingernail to snag and break the membranes at the back of the head. Peel them away from the baby's face as soon as the head emerges. Wipe the face and gently wipe away the mucus from around the baby's nose and mouth. If there is green meconium in the fluid around the baby, suction the mouth and nose with a soft rubber bulb syringe. **Note:** Be sure to expel air from the syringe first. Meconium is the waste matter (feces) of a newborn.

- Check Cord Around Neck. Check to see if the umbilical cord is wrapped around the baby's neck. If it is, carefully and quickly loosen the cord with your forefinger placed between the cord and the neck. If the cord is loose enough, slip it over the baby's head. Loosening the cord is necessary so that it will not choke the baby. **Caution:** Handle the cord carefully so it is not punctured or damaged in any way. It is still the lifeline for the baby.

  If the cord is wrapped around the neck too tightly and cannot be loosened, it must be tied off or clamped in two places and cut immediately. **Caution:** This should be done only if it is a life-threatening

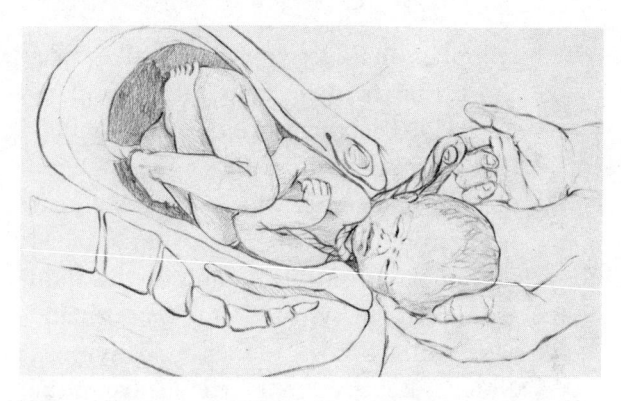

Fig. 7-2 Gently loosen cord from around the baby's neck with your forefinger while supporting the head with the other hand.

situation so be absolutely sure that the cord cannot be loosened and the baby is in trouble. (Procedure for cutting the cord is given on page 108.)

THE SHOULDERS AND BODY EMERGE

7. **Guide and Support.** The baby's head turns to face the mother's thigh in order to make delivery of the shoulders easier. Continue to support the head gently as the rest of the body is delivered. **Caution:** Do not pull or try to turn the baby's head as this may cause great harm to the baby. (Sometimes the head turns more slowly, along with the delivery of the shoulders.)

- After the head has been delivered, contractions usually stop for a few seconds then begin again. With the next contraction, tell the mother to bear down smoothly to deliver the upper shoulder. If the shoulders do not deliver after bearing down with two contractions, apply a gentle downward pressure on the baby's head to help deliver the upper shoulder, figure 7-3. **Caution:** Do not push the baby's head from side to side. Then gently raise the head to deliver the lower shoulder.

- After delivery of the shoulders, the rest of the body follows with a gush of fluid. Be prepared to receive the rest of the body as it may deliver quickly. **Caution:** The baby will be wet and slippery and may be difficult to hold. Keep a gentle support on the head as the body is delivered. As the feet are born, grasp the ankles firmly with one hand. Support the head with the other hand while you raise the baby's legs, figure 7-4. This position helps the mucus to drain, so the baby can breathe. The baby usually gives his first cry at this time. **Caution:** Hold the baby with its head down. Do not hold it in an upright position because mucus and secretions (which should drain out) will block the airway. Note the time of delivery. If someone else is near, ask him

96 LABOR AND DELIVERY

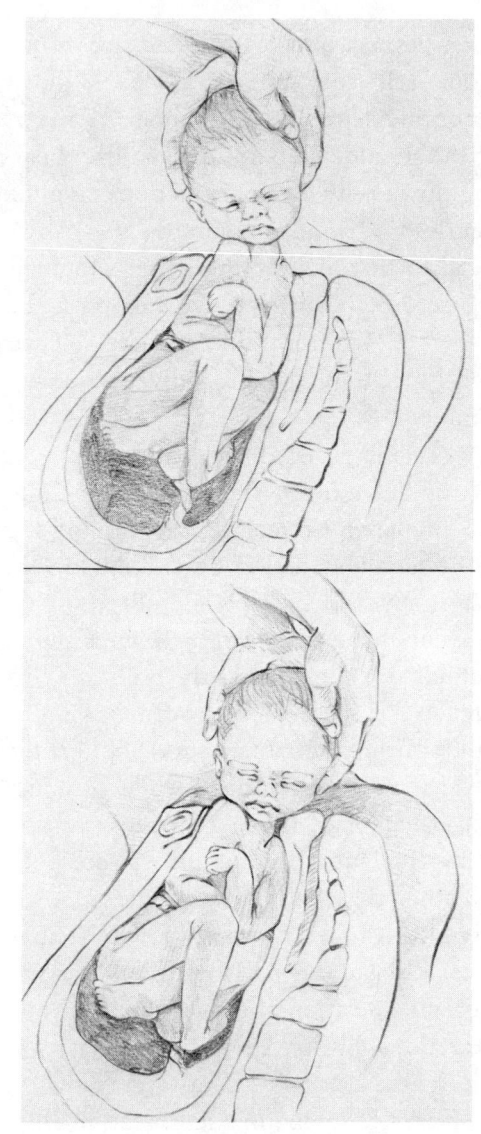

A. APPLY A GENTLE BUT FIRM DOWNWARD PRESSURE ON THE BABY'S HEAD TO HELP DELIVER THE UPPER SHOULDER.

B. THEN RAISE THE HEAD GENTLY TO DELIVER THE LOWER SHOULDER.

Fig. 7-3 Delivery of the shoulders

or her to check the time and write it down. **Caution**: Hold the baby firmly. Keep it close to the mother's body; the baby can be severely injured if it should fall or be dropped.

Dry the baby with a towel and place the baby, head down, on its side, between the mother's legs. The mother's body provides warmth for the baby and the

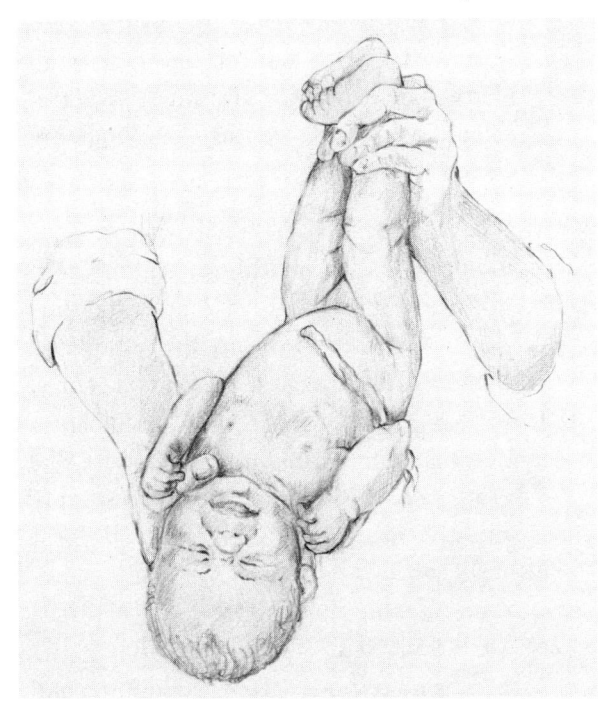

Fig. 7-4 After delivery, support the baby's head with one hand while you raise its legs in order to help mucus drain.

position helps to drain mucus. Wipe away remaining mucus. With your hand, gently stroke the baby's chest upward towards its mouth. Wipe away the mucus. Suction the mouth and nose with a bulb syringe to remove mucus, figure 7-5.

Check the heart beat. It should be about 100 beats a minute. If the heart rate is low, a vigorous massage with a dry towel will stimulate the baby. Keep the baby warm. Cover it with a towel or small blanket or article of clothing. Warmth, cleanliness, and gentle handling are essential to the newborn.

IF BABY FAILS TO BREATHE

If the baby is not breathing spontaneously within 30 seconds after delivery (about the time it takes to clear its airways) do the following:
- Rub baby's back or chest briskly but gently.
- If no response after 30 seconds, hold baby's ankles together with one hand. With the forefingers of the other hand, snap sharply against the soles of the baby's feet. Repeat after 30 seconds.
- If there is still no response, do artificial resuscitation, figure 7-6A, page 100.
- If there is no response after two minutes and you cannot locate a pulse, begin cardiopulmonary resuscitation, figure 7-6B, page 101.

EMERGENCY DELIVERY 99

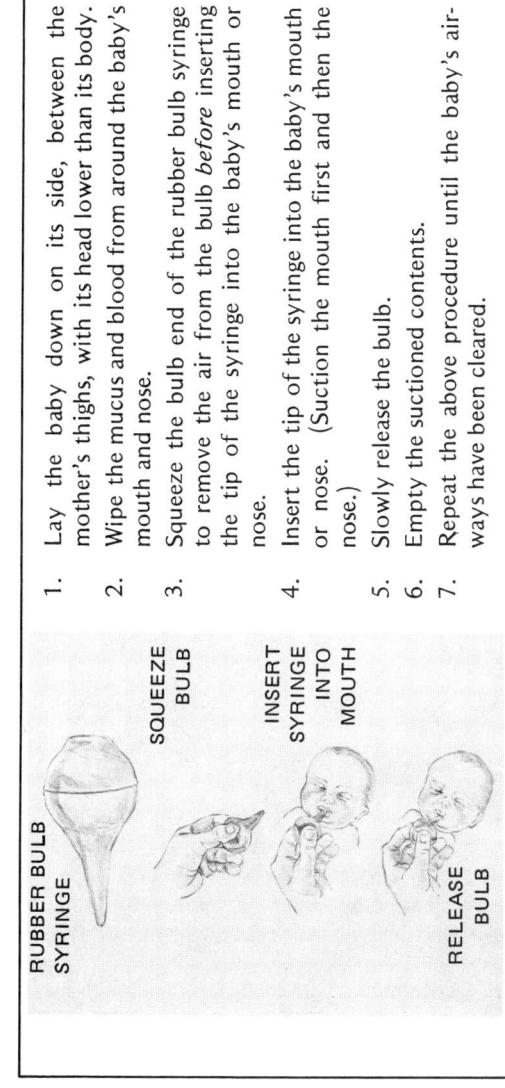

RUBBER BULB SYRINGE

SQUEEZE BULB

INSERT SYRINGE INTO MOUTH

RELEASE BULB

1. Lay the baby down on its side, between the mother's thighs, with its head lower than its body.
2. Wipe the mucus and blood from around the baby's mouth and nose.
3. Squeeze the bulb end of the rubber bulb syringe to remove the air from the bulb *before* inserting the tip of the syringe into the baby's mouth or nose.
4. Insert the tip of the syringe into the baby's mouth or nose. (Suction the mouth first and then the nose.)
5. Slowly release the bulb.
6. Empty the suctioned contents.
7. Repeat the above procedure until the baby's airways have been cleared.

CAUTION: Always squeeze the air from the bulb before inserting it into the baby's mouth or nose. This is necessary in order to prevent damaging the baby's lungs. Suctioning should only take about 30 seconds.

Fig. 7-5 The bulb syringe method of suctioning.

100 LABOR AND DELIVERY

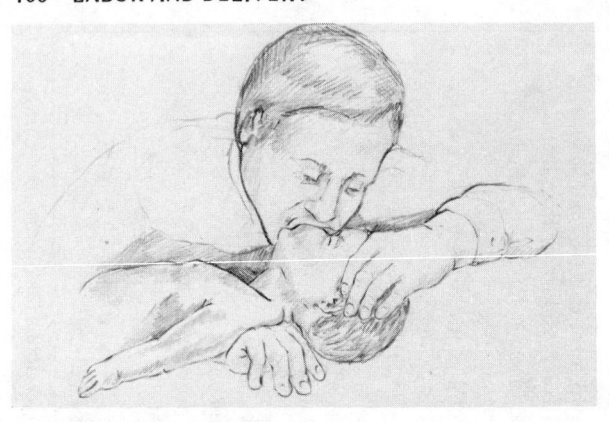

1. Clear the baby's mouth of any mucus.
2. Place your hand at base of the baby's neck in order to tilt its head back slightly. **CAUTION:** Tilting the baby's head too far may actually obstruct the baby's breathing passages.
3. Place your mouth over the baby's nose and mouth to create a tight seal.
4. Gently blow small puffs of air from your cheeks into the baby's nose and mouth (about one puff every 3 seconds).
5. After each puff, raise your mouth and turn your head to the side. This allows the air to escape back out of the baby's lungs and gives you a chance to take a breath. Be careful not to blow in air while the air is escaping.
6. Continue artificial breathing. Remember to use small, gentle puffs of air.
7. Observe for signs the baby is breathing on its own.

NOTE: The baby's chest should be rising and falling after each puff of air. If it is not, air is not going into the baby's lungs. Do the following:

- Be sure the baby's head is tilted far enough so the back of its tongue is not resting on the back of its throat. It may be necessary to pull the baby's jaw gently upward into a jutting position.
- Wipe or suction mucus from the baby's mouth; this may be blocking the baby's air passages.

Fig. 7-6A Mouth-to-mouth resuscitation of a newborn

EMERGENCY DELIVERY 101

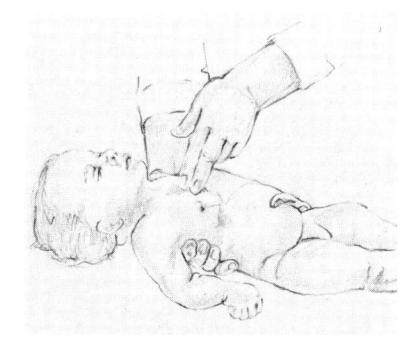

1. Locate the sternum. It is the plate of bone in the middle of the chest.

2. Place one hand under the baby's back.

3. With the tips of the index and middle fingers of the other hand, depress the midsternum about 1/2 to 3/4 inch.

4. Gently but forcibly do this at a rate of 80 to 100 compressions per minute (a little more than once per second). Pushing too hard can cause injury.

5. Give mouth-to-mouth resuscitation once after every 5 compressions. Do not interrupt the compressions while doing the mouth-to-mouth breathing.

ALTERNATE METHOD

1. Place both hands under the baby's back with thumbs meeting over the baby's sternum. Press down with both thumbs. Be gentle but firm.

2. Continue same as above.

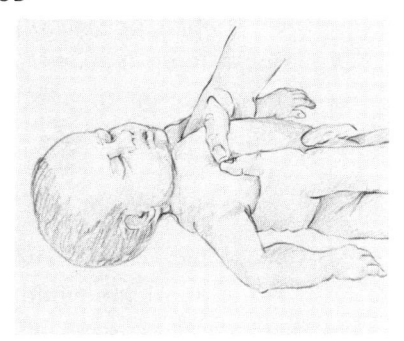

Fig. 7-6B Cardiopulmonary resuscitation of an infant

102 LABOR AND DELIVERY

Cardiopulmonary resuscitation is the combination of artificial respiration (mouth-to-mouth breathing) and manual circulation (closed chest massage).

Note: Newborns have been known to revive even after 20 minutes of continued resuscitation without damage to the brain; don't give up hope.

THE PLACENTA AND THE CORD

There will be a lull in the contractions before the placenta is delivered. Keep the baby on its side with the head slightly lower than the body. Watch frequently to be sure it continues to breathe without difficulty. It is not necessary to cut the umbilical cord unless medical care cannot be obtained for several hours. Because of the danger of infection through the open end of the cord if it is cut with unsterile equipment, it is better to leave the cord uncut. However, it may be clamped or tied off while waiting for the placenta to be expelled. **Caution:** If you do not clamp or tie off the cord, remember to hold the placenta above the baby.

DELIVERY OF THE PLACENTA

1. **Check and Massage Uterus.** Place a hand on the mother's abdomen to check the height and consistency of the fundus (top of the uterus). After the baby has been

delivered, the uterus should contract; it is usually felt at the level of the navel (belly button) or slightly below. Firmness of the uterus means that the blood vessels are closed off and excess bleeding is prevented. Massage the uterus until it feels hard and firm, figure 7-8, page 106.

2. **Wait For Signs**. Watch for signs that the placenta has separated from the wall of the uterus. These signs usually appear about 5 to 20 minutes after delivery of the baby:

- The umbilical cord (still attached to the placenta) advances about 3 or more inches farther out of the vagina.
- A trickle or sudden spurt of blood flows from the vagina. This is due to the separating of the placenta from the wall of the uterus.
- The uterus feels like a round ball and usually becomes more firm.

Never attempt to deliver the placenta before it separates from the wall of the uterus; this can be dangerous to the life of the mother and baby.

3. **Check Firmness of Uterus**. If firm, ask the mother to bear down to expel the placenta. If it is not firm, massage it until it remains firm. If the uterus is not firm, it may turn inside out, causing a very grave complication known as inversion of the uterus.

4. **Receive the Placenta.** Hold a container just below the vaginal opening to receive the placenta. Keep the placenta close to the vulva until all the afterbirth has been delivered. This prevents tearing of the membranes before they have separated completely from the wall of the uterus.

   When the placenta is expelled, it is accompanied by bleeding. Bleeding may be moderate or excessive. If the bleeding is moderate, simply place a sanitary napkin, diaper, folded towel, or clean cloth against the mother's perineum.

5. **Aftercare.** After delivery of the placenta, the uterus should feel like a firm, round mass below the navel and remain this way. It should be checked about every 5 minutes for the first hour after delivery to make sure it remains firm. If the uterus relaxes (feels soft and limp), it must be massaged until it is firm again. This is essential in order to prevent hemorrhaging. **Caution**: As soon as the uterus is firm, discontinue the massage. The uterus should only be massaged when and if it becomes soft and limp. Unnecessary massage of the uterus when it is firm can actually make it relax. Also, unnecessary massage makes the woman uncomfortable.

EMERGENCY DELIVERY 105

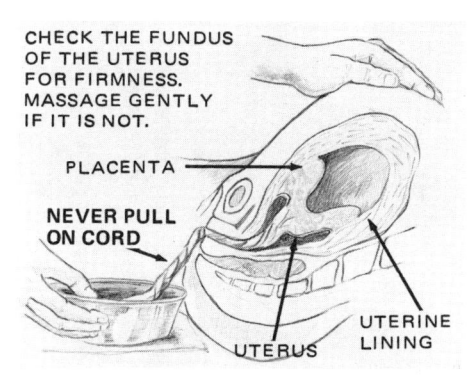

(Figure illustration: CHECK THE FUNDUS OF THE UTERUS FOR FIRMNESS. MASSAGE GENTLY IF IT IS NOT. PLACENTA. NEVER PULL ON CORD. UTERUS. UTERINE LINING.)

Fig. 7-7 The afterbirth or placenta usually delivers without help.

Put the placenta in a towel, plastic bag, or other container. It must be transported to the hospital with the mother. The placenta is examined by a doctor in order to determine if all the afterbirth has been delivered. Any part of the placenta that remains in the mother may cause serious complications. Remember that the placenta must be placed higher than the baby if the umbilical cord has not been tied off. If the placenta is still attached to the baby, place the wrapped placenta next to the baby and wrap them both in a blanket. Otherwise the placenta may fall and tear the cord.

IF THE PLACENTA FAILS TO DELIVER

If medical help cannot be obtained shortly and the placenta cannot be delivered by the

106 LABOR AND DELIVERY

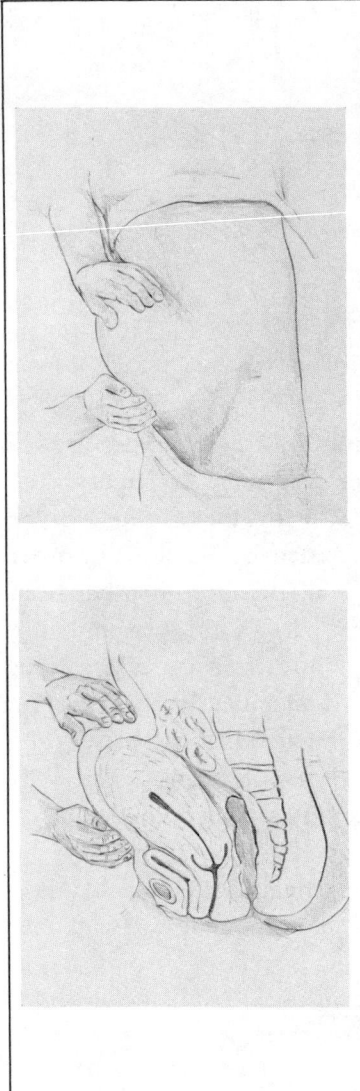

1. Locate fundus (top) of uterus. It may appear as a grapefruit-size protrusion in the area of the mother's navel.
2. Place one hand around the fundus of the uterus. Fingers should be deep into the abdomen behind the fundus; the thumbs should rest on the top of the fundus.
3. Place the other hand on the mother's abdomen just above the pubic bone. This hand is used only to support the uterus. Do not massage or apply pressure with this hand.
4. Massage the fundus of the uterus vigorously with a circular motion until it becomes firm.
   Caution: DO NOT SQUEEZE THE UTERUS.

Fig. 7-8 Proper way to massage the uterus.

mother's bearing down, do the following:

- Make sure the uterus is firm by continuing to massage.
- Cup your hand around the fundus of the uterus.
- Exert a steady, gentle pressure on the fundus, pushing it in the direction of the vagina. This should move the placenta out of the vagina. **Caution:** Do not squeeze the uterus. This procedure must be done *gently* and must *never* be done unless the uterus is firm. Do not push hard on the uterus and never pull on the umbilical cord.

IF THERE IS EXCESSIVE BLEEDING

If the bleeding is excessive (more than two cups) it is considered hemorrhage. Do the following:

- Massage the uterus until it feels firm.
- If hemorrhage does not stop from massaging the uterus, place towels or clean cloths over the vagina and perineum.
- Cross the woman's legs tightly.
- Elevate the lower half of her body.
- Encourage the baby to nurse. This helps the uterus to contract and reduces bleeding.
- Seek medical help immediately.

THE CORD

Do not be in a hurry to *cut* the cord. It is better to wait for sterilized equipment if none is available; a severe infection may result from cutting the cord with an unsterile instrument. Also, if there is doubt about the procedure, the cord may be left attached to the baby and taken to the hospital. However, the cord may be clamped or tied off. This can be done either after the baby is born or after the placenta has been delivered. If you should wait until the placenta has been delivered before clamping or tying off the cord, remember to keep the placenta higher than the baby.

To clamp or tie off the cord, you will need alcohol and sterile clamps or ties which have been boiled (and have not been touched).

1. Place the baby on its side on a clean towel.
2. Wait until the cord has stopped beating. Feel it with your hand until it is no longer pulsating (usually about 30 to 60 seconds after the baby's birth).
3. Handle the cord carefully to prevent tearing or damaging it. If the cord is damaged before it is tied off, the baby could bleed to death.
4. If available, use an antiseptic such as alcohol to clean the cord. Vinegar may be used if alcohol is not available.

5. Use two sterile clamps or two white cotton tapes, strips of cloth, flat shoelaces, or pieces of heavy twine. The ties should be about 12 inches long. **Caution:** Never use thread or string or thin materials; they will cut through the cord while you are tightening the knot. (Materials should have been boiled beforehand. Bring water to a boil, drop in the ties and boil for 20 minutes. There is no need to dry the ties.)
6. Use a square knot to tie the cord. Tie the knots slowly but be sure each is tight. Avoid a rapid pull on the ties.
7. Tie the cord in two places. First tie about 4 to 6 inches from the baby's belly button; then leave a space of one or two inches and tie again. (It is better to leave too much next to the baby than not enough.)

To cut the cord, *after you have tied it off* as described, continue as follows:

- Be sure cord is not pulsating.
- Use sterile scissors or a new single-edge razor blade.
- The cutting instrument must be sterile. If sterile scissors are not available, drop the open scissors into boiling water. Be sure the scissors are covered by the water and the blades are sterilized. Cover and boil for 20 minutes. (The scissors and tapes can be

110 LABOR AND DELIVERY

A. TIE THE CORD (OR CLAMP IT) ABOUT 4 TO 6 INCHES FROM THE NAVEL. TIE (CLAMP) AGAIN ABOUT 2 INCHES FROM THE FIRST ONE.

B. HOW TO TIE A SQUARE KNOT

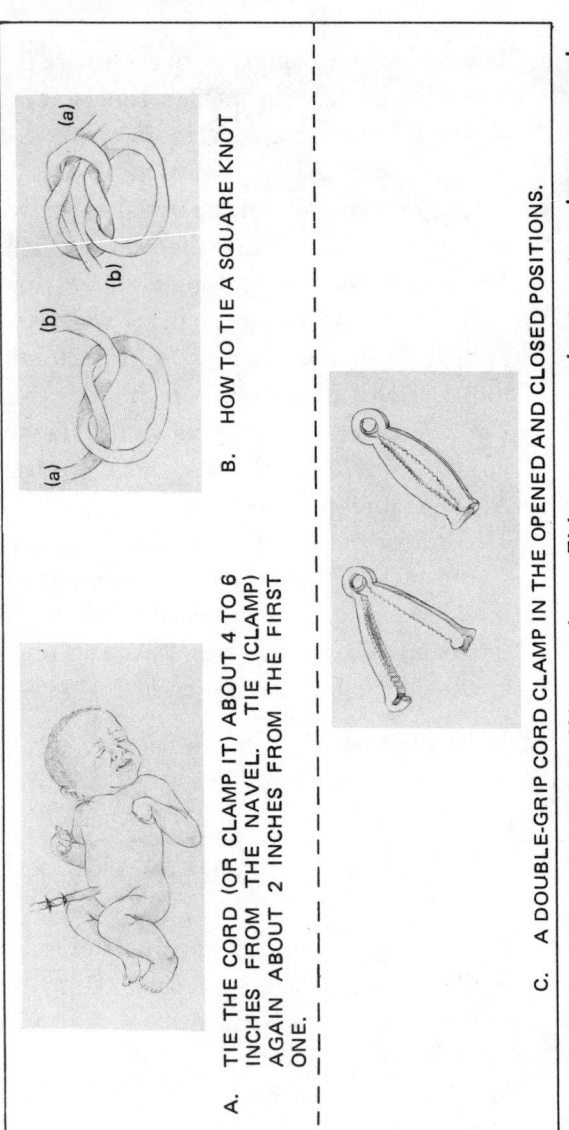

C. A DOUBLE-GRIP CORD CLAMP IN THE OPENED AND CLOSED POSITIONS.

Fig. 7-9 The umbilical cord is tied off in two places. Either two square knots or two clamps are used.

boiled together beforehand.) After boiling, the water can be drained off and the scissors left in the covered pan until ready for use.
- Cut the cord *between the two ties*.
- After cutting the cord between the two ties, check the ends for bleeding.
- Periodically check the end of the cord which is attached to the baby. If there is any sign of bleeding, tie the cord again — a short distance from the first tie, that is, between the baby's belly button and the old first tie.

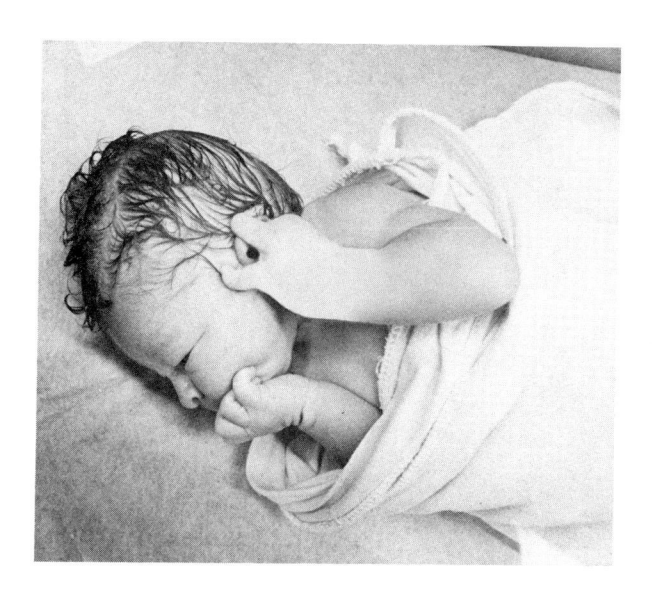

Fig. 7-10 The newborn often assumes the fetal position immediately after delivery.

112 LABOR AND DELIVERY

Do not attempt to tighten the original tie. If the cord is not closed off completely, the baby may bleed to death. After the cord has been cut, wrap the baby in a blanket and give it to the mother to hold. If the cord has only been clamped or tied off, it will be necessary to wait for the placenta to be delivered before letting the mother hold her child. If there is any danger of the mother and baby being separated, be sure to identify the baby. The name of the mother and father, the sex of the baby, the date, time, and place of the birth should be included in the identification.

-8-
Complications and Unusual Deliveries

About 85 percent of all births are normal deliveries. However some situations do occur that can threaten the life of both the mother and baby. Observation, reporting, technical skill, physical and emotional supportive measures must all be carried out with a fine degree of competence. Yet, in a situation of stress, where the labor and delivery process is complicated, even more is demanded of the person in attendance. Two critical points must be considered whenever something is wrong with the labor or delivery process:

- Obtain medical help as soon as possible.
- Give supportive care to the woman in labor.

The necessity to reach medical help is of utmost importance for the expectant mother and the baby's well-being. This is especially true when the fetus is in an abnormal position such as: an ROP or LOP position, shoulder presentation, face and brow (forehead) presentations. In most of these cases there is nothing else one can do but talk to the expectant mother, and give her as much physical and emotional comfort as possible while getting her to the hospital or doctor.

Premature labor and prolonged labor may present complications. Therefore the technician must be knowledgeable about normal delivery so he can be ready to handle the unexpected complication. Sometimes an expectant mother goes into labor before the baby is due. A newborn is said to be a premature baby if it is born 3 or more weeks before the expected date of birth.

Occasionally, one might observe a woman in labor for hours and hours without any apparent progress. The cause of difficult labor may be related to three factors: the forces, the passage, or the passenger. The forces refers to the uterus and its contractions; the passage refers to the structures that make up the birth canal; the passenger refers to the fetus.

A delay in any of the stages could be due to the uterine contractions being of poor quality or due to maternal exhaustion. The actual reason for the failure of the uterus to contract enough is not known. Some contributing factors, however, may be: age of the mother; a rigid, tight cervix; an oversize baby which has overdistended the uterus; and others.

If the expectant mother is having contractions every 2 or 3 minutes, birth will probably take place shortly. If, however, labor does not progress and the baby's head or a presenting part is not visible in 20 minutes, this would indicate that all is not well. Medical help is necessary so the woman should be taken to the hospital without any further delay. If labor goes on too long, the baby may be injured or die and the mother can become exhausted and dehydrated. Therefore, it is obvious that prevention is the best way of avoiding any of these serious outcomes. The woman in labor must be closely observed; frequency, duration, and intensity of the contractions must be noted and reported to the doctor in order to prevent harm to the mother or child.

Sometimes the pelvis is too small for the baby to pass through. Other complications which may require inducing of labor by the doctor are: diabetes, heart disease, kidney disease, premature rupture of the membranes, and premature separation of the placenta. The doctor may hasten the labor by giving medication to the expectant mother, using forceps, or performing a cesarean section to deliver the baby through an incision in the abdomen and wall of the uterus.

If the patient has been under medical care, some of these conditions are foreseen and plans are made for hospitalization before labor starts. However, sometimes the complication is not expected or the mother-to-be has not had prenatal care. The technician or attendant may find an emergency situation on hand. In such cases, the technician can only give much-needed comfort and get the maternity patient to the hospital right away. Remember this is a frightening time for the expectant mother — be sure she is not left alone. Bewilderment and fright may be overwhelming; she may not be able to handle the situation because of physical discomfort as well as fear. If someone is concerned about her, she will be better able to relax and cooperate so that additional complications can be avoided and the present situation be brought under control.

> Signs that may indicate labor is not progressing normally are:
>
> - Abnormal vaginal bleeding
> - Contractions stop after labor has begun
> - Rise in blood pressure
> - A rigid uterus after a contraction is over
> - Severe headache and dizziness
> - Passage of meconium-stained fluid (unless baby is in breech position)
> - Umbilical cord can be seen

Complications and unusual deliveries to be covered in this chapter are: premature births;

breech births and other abnormal fetal positions; prolapsed umbilical cord; multiple births; miscarriage or abortion; and the stillborn.

PREMATURE BIRTH

If the baby is born 3 or more weeks before the expected date of birth, it is said to be premature. Although only 7 to 10 percent of all live births are premature, prematurity is the most frequent cause of death in infants. The premature baby needs special care if it is to survive.

The premature baby appears to be listless and inactive. It is much smaller and thinner than a full-term baby. It weighs less than 5 1/2 pounds and is less than 18 inches in length. The head is quite large in proportion to the body. The fontanels (soft spots) of the head are large and the lines of closure (sutures) are quite prominent. The cry is feeble, and the sucking reflex is poor or absent. The tiny features are sharp and angular. The skin is wrinkled, dull red, and covered with fine downy hair. Respirations are quite irregular. Body temperature is unstable and below normal, often 34° to 36° Celsius (94° to 96°F). The blood vessels are very thin and fragile. Many premature babies are unable to swallow. If the baby is premature, focus your efforts on: (1) helping the baby breathe, (2) keeping it warm, (3) handling it with care, and (4) preventing infection.

118 LABOR AND DELIVERY

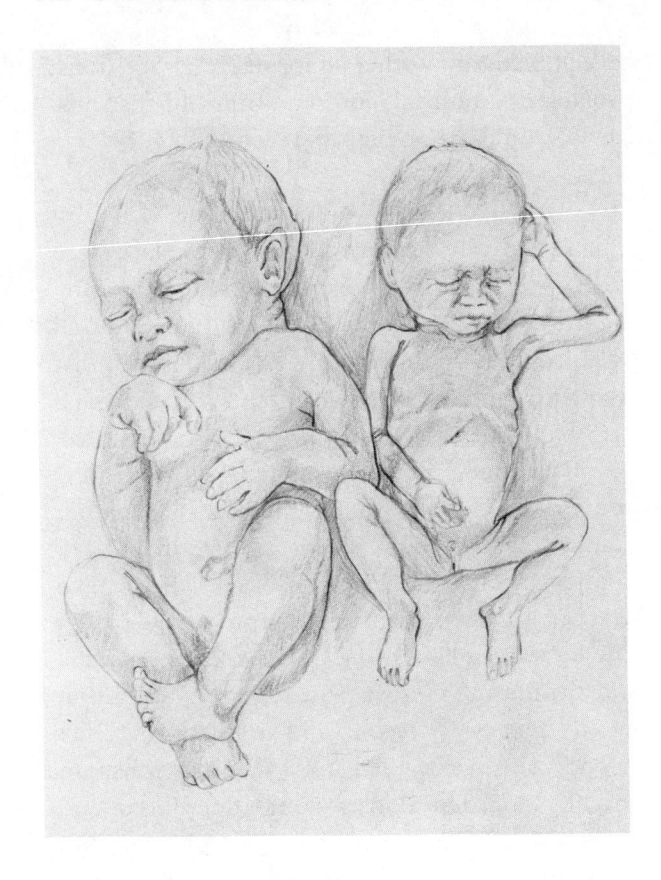

Fig. 8-1 The premature infant usually weighs under 2.5 kilograms (5 1/2 pounds). Because of lack of fat, the baby has thinner arms and legs, thinner cheeks and chin, a large head and large abdomen. The skin is loose and wrinkled and the baby looks old and anxious.

Help Baby Breathe

1. Establish the baby's breathing. Gentle stimulation such as wiggling a foot or stroking the chest upward (while the baby is being held with its head down) may get the infant started. **Caution:** Do not hold it in an upright position after birth because mucus and secretions which should drain out may block the airway. Since lung tissue of a premature baby is frequently not fully developed, the lungs may not be able to fully expand. Use gentle suction, if bulb syringe is available, to keep the mouth and nose clear of mucus.

2. **Administer oxygen if needed.** Not all premature infants need oxygen but some do. Giving oxygen to a premature infant may have certain dangers. However, if the oxygen is administered indirectly and gently, in low concentration (40%) for a short period of time, the benefits outweigh the dangers.

   - Do not give oxygen for longer than 15 to 20 minutes. Limit the concentration to 40%. **Caution:** Avoid prolonged use or high concentrations of oxygen. Too much oxygen can cause blindness.
   - Keep the head extended. Be sure the baby's chin is not resting on the chest.

This position can obstruct the airway and restrict the flow of air into the lungs.

- Make a "tent" over the baby's head with newspaper, aluminum foil or whatever material is available. Allow the oxygen to enter the tent in a slow, gentle stream. Aim the stream of oxygen towards the top of the tent. **Caution:** Never allow the oxygen to blow directly on the baby's face or into its eyes. Never use regular equipment that is part of the oxygen tank setup; it is too large and forceful for administering oxygen to any infant.

Keep Baby Warm and Handle With Care

The premature infant cannot shiver or perspire. The tiny body has no way of adjusting to the temperature of the environment. Since the lung tissue is also immature and incapable of expanding fully, respiratory diseases such as pneumonia, bronchitis, and other lung disorders are likely to occur if the baby is allowed to be chilled.

- Wrap the infant snugly in a warm blanket or article of clothing. With the cord tied off, wrap the baby and the placenta in the blanket.

- If available, wrap aluminum foil or newspaper over the blanket, around the baby. This helps to maintain the body heat. **Caution:** Be careful not to cover the baby's face.
- Place the baby in a warm spot (90° Fahrenheit or 32° Celsius) with its head lower than its body: this will help the mucus to drain.

The premature is very fragile and can bruise very easily. Do not handle him any more than is absolutely necessary. The premature baby cannot afford to lose even the slightest bit of blood. Therefore it is best not to cut the umbilical cord unless it is absolutely necessary.

If the cord has stopped pulsating, the cord may be tied off with two ties as described on page 108. Note: Remember to keep the placenta higher than the baby if the cord is not tied or cut. (If the cord is cut, check it often for any sign of bleeding; if bleeding is present, tie the cord again close to the first tie. See page 110 and figure 7-9.)

Prevent Infection

The body defenses are not fully developed so the premature baby cannot fight off infections. The premature baby is easily infected. Any infection becomes a serious threat to the baby's life.

- Keep the baby away from other people as much as possible.
- Do not breathe directly on the baby's face, unless mouth-to-mouth resuscitation is essential for its survival. A lightweight gauze may be used if it is available.

BREECH BIRTHS

If the buttocks of the baby or the baby's feet are visible at the vaginal opening instead of the head, a breech birth will be taking place. Breech births occur in about 3 percent of all term deliveries. A breech birth may be suspected if black, tar-colored matter is seen coming out of the vagina. This is meconium, the contents of the baby's bowel. Upon seeing meconium, it is necessary to check the vaginal opening to be sure that the baby is really in breech presentation because — although it is normal for meconium to be present when the buttocks or feet are there — it is not normal if the head is at the vaginal opening. (In such a case, the baby is in trouble and needs medical attention.)

There are three classifications of breech presentation: (1) complete — the buttocks and feet present and the knees are drawn up, (2) footling — one or both feet present, and (3) frank — the buttocks present and the legs are extended up and against the abdomen and chest. The most common is a frank presentation.

FRANK BREECH

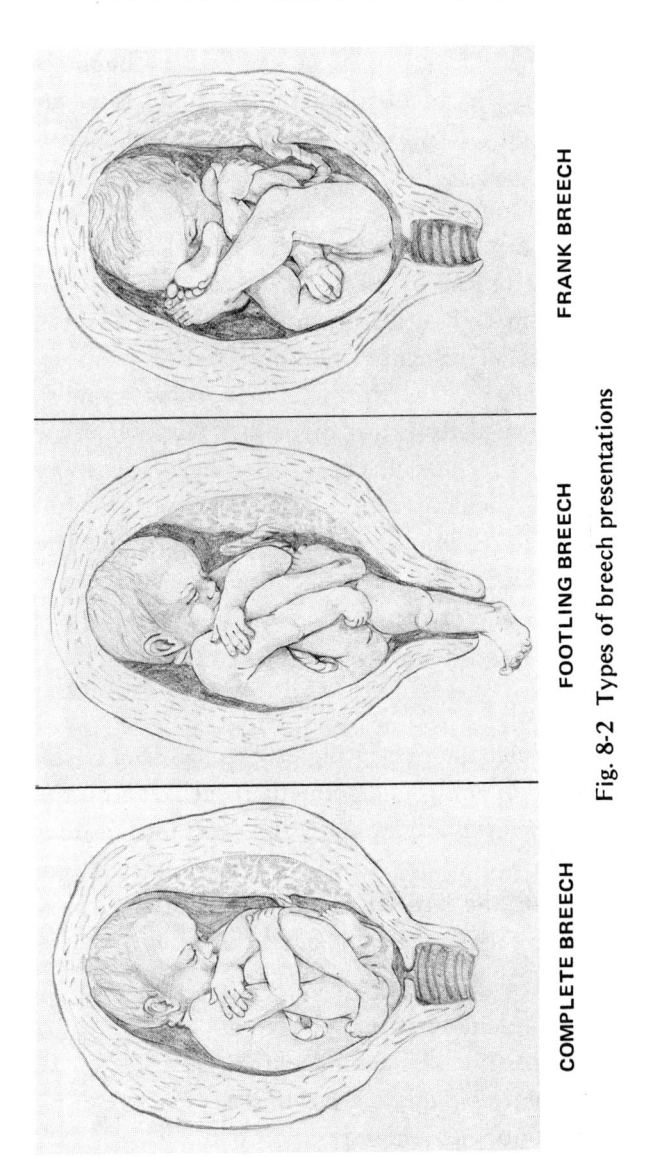

FOOTLING BREECH

COMPLETE BREECH

Fig. 8-2 Types of breech presentations

The delivery of breech positioned babies is usually spontaneous and the outcome is generally good. However, it does involve more risk to the infant than a head presentation. The danger comes from the trauma of delivery and the chance of a prolapsed cord. Also, labor is usually longer for a breech delivery. Therefore, more time is available to get the woman to a hospital. This should be done if at all possible. If, however, the birth is happening rapidly, delivery usually is not difficult. This is because a rapid breech delivery usually means the baby is small, the contractions are strong and forceful, and there is ample room in the birth canal. The baby will probably deliver spontaneously with little need of assistance.

Preparation for Breech Delivery

When the presenting part can be seen at the vaginal opening and immediate delivery of the baby is inevitable, prepare the expectant mother as you would for any delivery. Details were given in the preceding chapter. Briefly, they include these considerations:

- Provide privacy
- Explain what you plan to do
- Position the woman (firm surface, knees bent, legs apart, head raised)
- Drape her properly

COMPLICATIONS AND UNUSUAL DELIVERIES

- Scrub your hands and arms thoroughly
- Comfort and reassure the expectant mother

When delivering a baby in breech position, focus your attention on: (1) guiding and supporting the emerging infant, (2) helping the baby breathe, (3) handling it with care, (4) preventing infection in the mother and the child, and (5) reassuring the mother.

The presenting part of a breech presentation is usually the buttocks, so part of the buttocks will be seen at the beginning of the second stage of labor. At first it will be visible only at the height of each contraction. Gradually more and more of the baby's buttocks will be seen until the mother's perineum and anus are stretched to the point where — due to the pressure — the buttocks bulge outward.

PART OF THE BUTTOCKS IS SEEN

Work with Contractions. Allow the baby to deliver spontaneously as a result of the mother's bearing-down efforts.

Prevent Infection. Do not touch the mother's perineum or the baby. If the contents of the lower bowel are expelled, wipe the feces away from the mother's rectum (toward her back). If your hands touch the feces, scrub them over again with soap and water. Since the delivery

126 LABOR AND DELIVERY

may be a quick one and you need the time, avoid touching the feces.

Reassure and Inform. Remind the mother to keep her thighs and pelvic floor as relaxed as possible and keep her informed of the progress.

Discourage Pushing. Promote Breathing. As the buttocks are about to emerge, breathing exercises will help to slow down delivery and lessen the risk of tearing the delicate tissues of the mother's perineum.

BUTTOCKS AND TRUNK EMERGE

Guide and Support. Do not allow the baby to pop out.

- Support the baby with the palm of your hand as the buttocks and trunk of the

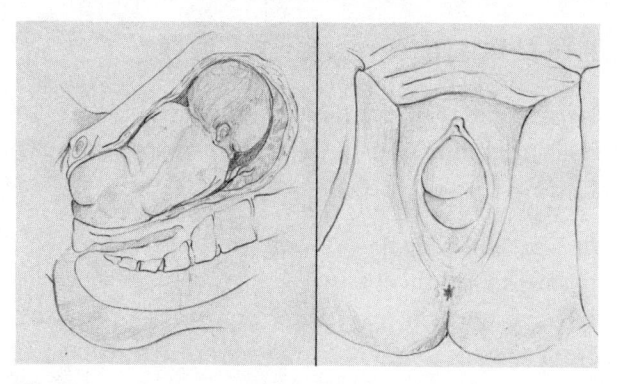

Fig. 8-3 As breech labor proceeds, the presenting buttocks become more visible.

COMPLICATIONS AND UNUSUAL DELIVERIES 127

baby emerge from the vagina. After the trunk is delivered, the legs will descend.
- Grasp the ankles with one hand while supporting the body with the other hand.

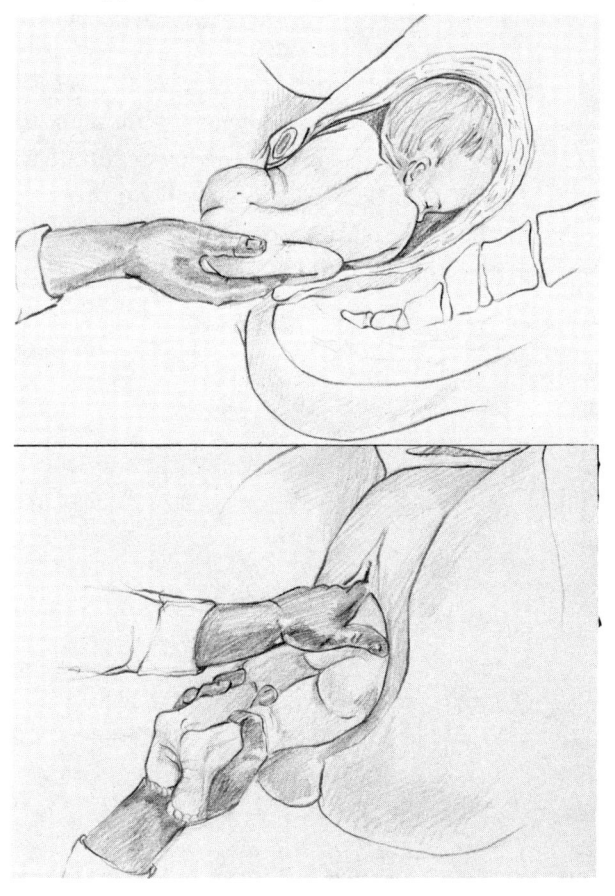

Fig. 8-4 Guide and support the emerging buttocks, trunk, and ankles.

THE SHOULDERS

Guide and Support. Ask the woman to bear down hard with the contractions in order to expel the shoulders.

- If bearing down does not deliver the shoulders and arms, gently raise the baby's body towards the woman's abdomen to assist in the delivery of the lower shoulder.
- Apply a gentle but firm downward pressure to the baby's body to assist in the delivery of the upper shoulder.

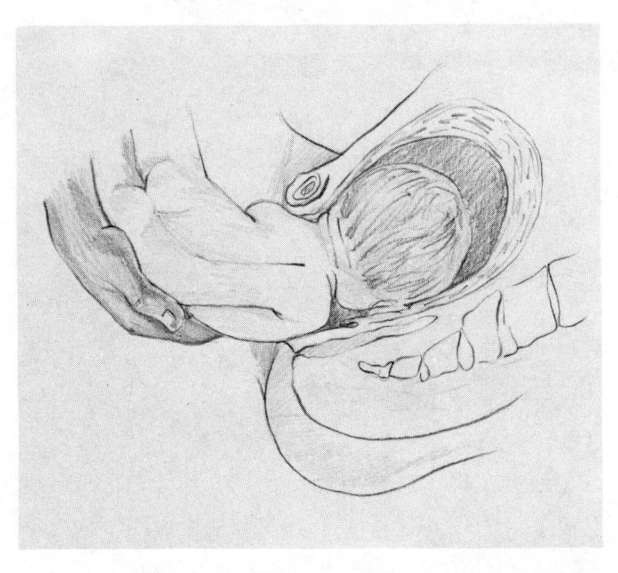

Fig. 8-5 To help the lower shoulder deliver, prepare to gently insert the first and middle finger over the baby's lower shoulder and raise the body upward.

THE ARMS

Guide and Support. Usually, the arms deliver after the shoulders as normally, they are folded across the chest while the baby is in the uterus. The arms should deliver before the head does. Therefore if the arms are above the head, they must be brought out before the head is delivered.

- Gently insert your first and middle fingers into the mother's vagina over the baby's lower shoulder up to the baby's upper arm. The arm which is most posterior (that would be the one closest to the mother's back) is withdrawn first because there is more room in that part of the birth canal.

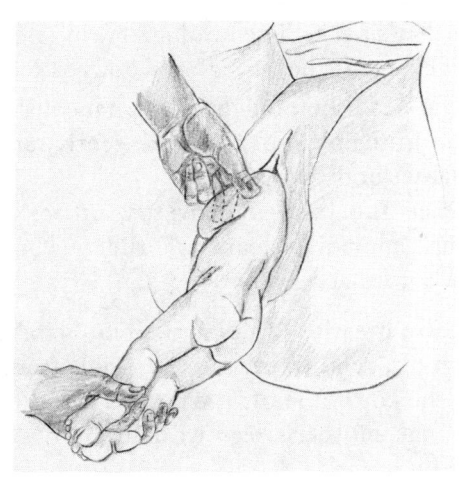

Fig. 8-6 Use the sides of the fingers against the baby's arm to bring it down and out of the vagina.

LABOR AND DELIVERY

- Using the sides of your fingers along the length of the baby's upper arm, gently bring the arm down across its face and chest and out of the vagina. **Caution:** Be sure to use the sides of your fingers. Pulling the arm by using the crook of your finger may break the baby's delicate bone.
- Lower the baby's body and extract the anterior arm in the same manner: insert your fingers over the baby's upper shoulder and gently bring the arm down and out of the the vagina.

THE HEAD

Guide and Support. After the shoulders and arms deliver, the baby rotates spontaneously so it faces the mother's back. The head is now in a position to be delivered; the rest of the body is outside.

- The head should deliver spontaneously. To aid in the birth of the head, gently raise the baby's body upward.
- Once the head is delivered, proceed with the immediate care of the newborn as in a normal delivery (pages 95-98).

Help Baby Breathe. As described in the preceding chapter, remove mucus and fluids (suction). Check the cord. Tie off the cord. Place the baby against the mother's legs with its head slightly lowered.

- If there are respiratory problems, start cardiopulmonary resuscitation, pages 100-101.

Delivery of the placenta and the immediate care of the mother were described fully in the preceding chapter. Briefly, they are:
- (a) Place a container next to the mother's vulva to catch the placenta.
- (b) Wrap the baby and the placenta together in a blanket.
- (c) Check mother's bleeding. Apply a pad against the vulva.
- (d) Identify the baby — record the parents' names, baby's sex, date, time and place of birth.
- (e) Place the baby in the mother's arms and keep them both warm and comfortable until arrival at the hospital.

IF THE HEAD DOES NOT DELIVER WITHIN 3 MINUTES

Rest the baby on the palm of your hand, with its legs straddling your forearm.
- Insert two fingers in the vagina and place them gently in the baby's mouth. With the fingertips, gently bend the baby's chin down on its chest. This places the head in a position where it can be more easily expelled. DO NOT PULL or use force. Sterile gloves should be used when available.
- Apply firm downward pressure on the mother's abdomen to help expel the head. **Caution**: Do not pull the baby. Pulling

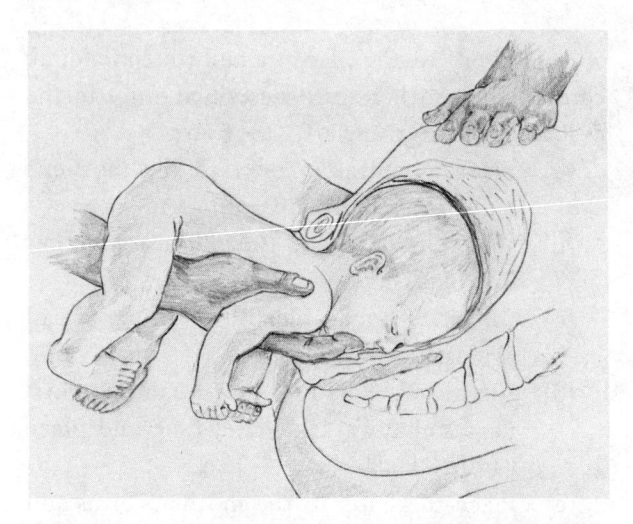

Fig. 8-7 If the head does not deliver after the baby has rotated and is facing the mother's back, two fingers may be inserted to pull the lower jaw down and so bend the head; at the same time firm downward pressure is applied to the woman's abdomen. DO NOT PULL the baby out.

may permanently damage the baby's spinal cord, nerves, and/or breathing organs.

IF THE HEAD STILL DOES NOT DELIVER

Create and maintain an air passage to the baby's nose so the infant will not suffocate:

- Move the two fingers towards the baby's face.
- Press the wall of the vagina away from the baby's face with the back of your fingers.
- Form a "V" by placing your fingers at each side of the baby's nose.

COMPLICATIONS AND UNUSUAL DELIVERIES 133

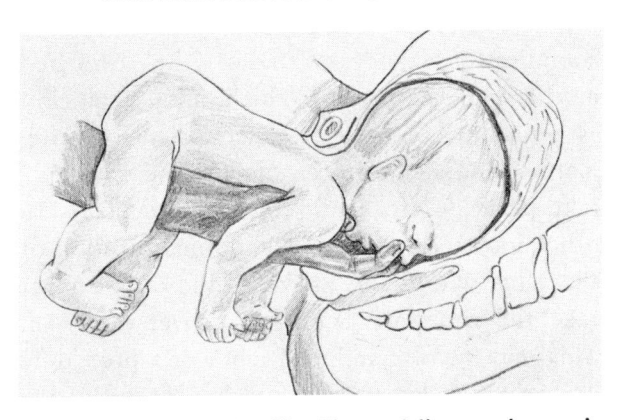

Fig. 8-8 If the head will still not deliver, make an air passage. With two fingers, form a "V" around the baby's nose. Press the back of the fingers against the vaginal wall so there is room for the baby to breathe until medical help arrives.

The baby can breathe with this assistance until the head is delivered, or until medical help arrives.

ABNORMAL FETAL POSITIONS

Some abnormal fetal positions are more complicated than others. When emergency medical technicians, law enforcement officers, and firefighters develop skills, they may feel confident enough to intervene if the woman's life is in danger and no medical help is available. However, this text is not meant to replace classroom instruction or medical supervision. Its purpose is to inform and to supplement such instruction. Therefore, in cases of unusual complications and deliveries, the expected mother must be taken to the hospital as quickly as possible. In some instances — such as premature labors and breech birth — the birth may take place before medical help is available. In other instances — such as abnormal position of the fetus within the uterus — the doctor must take the necessary action to deliver the child. This may involve induced labor or a procedure known as a "version," a turning around of the baby while it is in the uterus. Needless to say, this requires extraordinary knowledge and skill.

Shoulder, Face and Brow Presentations

Shoulder presentations are seen in about 1 out of 200 cases. The infant lies crosswise in the mother's pelvis. If labor sets in while the child is in this position, there is danger to the mother and the child; it may cause a rupture of the uterus and also places more stress on the infant. If the mother has been under the doctor's care, this complication may be foreseen. It will be necessary for the doctor to intervene by trying to turn the baby while it is still in the uterus. He does this by bringing one foot or both feet down into the vagina and delivers the baby in this footling breech position.

Face presentations are also seen about once in every 200 cases. The infant's face is often

COMPLICATIONS AND UNUSUAL DELIVERIES 135

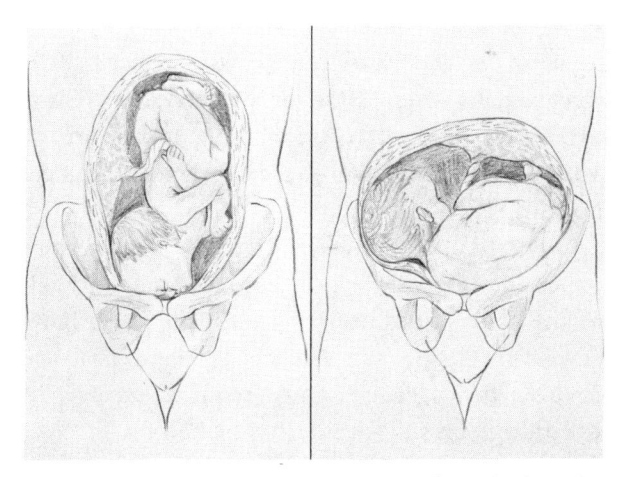

Fig. 8-9 Delivery becomes more complicated when the presenting part is a face or shoulder.

swollen and purplish due to birth trauma. Brow (forehead) presentations are even more rare and are harder to deliver because the largest diameter of the baby's head is presenting.

Persistent Occiput Posterior Positions

This position prolongs labor as the fetal head enters the pelvis with the head (occiput) directed diagonally posterior (ROP or LOP position). Under the circumstances, the head must rotate through an arc of 135 degrees in the process of internal rotation rather than the normal 90 degree arc. With good contractions, adequate flexion and an average size baby, most of these occiput posterior positioned babies will spontaneously rotate through the 135 degree arc as soon as the head reaches the pelvic floor. Occasionally these ROP or LOP babies do not make the internal rotation through the arc of 135 degrees and will be born with the face upward.

It should be noted that the mother may experience a great deal of discomfort in her back as the baby's head presses against the lower back (sacrum) during the rotation. Hand pressure against the sacrum, and frequent change of position from side to side can be helpful.

PROLAPSED UMBILICAL CORD

If the umbilical cord can be seen beside the baby as it appears at the vaginal opening, or if the cord is seen coming out of the vaginal opening, it is called a *prolapsed cord*. This is not a common complication; it happens only about once out of every 400 births. It is however, a very serious complication because of the high infant death rate associated with it. The threat to the baby's life is caused by the cord being pressed between the baby and the mother's bony pelvis. This shuts off the baby's blood supply from the cord and, with it, the baby's oxygen supply. The baby quickly suffocates.

- Check the cord to see if it is pulsating. If the cord is pulsating, the baby is still alive. Prolapse of the cord is an emergency situation and the importance of supportive care cannot be overemphasized. Medical help should be obtained quickly. In the meantime, it is important to remember that the objective is to relieve pressure on the cord and protect it from injury.

- Raise the hips higher than the rest of the body. Compression of the cord is relieved because the baby's head is not pressing as strongly against the cord and the vaginal opening. However, this is only a temporary measure; medical attention must be obtained promptly.
- Protect the cord in a warm, moist towel.

Elevate The Hips

As soon as the cord is discovered at the vaginal opening, gently place the woman in a knee-chest position. Gather pillows, blankets, or whatever is available to provide elevation and support. The knee-chest position is uncomfortable and the woman will soon tire. Place the pillows next to her and help her turn on her side so that her hips are higher than her chest and she is in a side-lying position. This is more comfortable and helps to keep pressure off the cord while waiting for medical attention.

Comfort and Reassure

Cover the woman with a blanket to keep her warm. If oxygen is available, administer small amounts to her. This will help to increase the oxygen supply to the baby and the expectant mother.

Remember to change the woman's position in a slow, gentle manner. Be calm, efficient, and reassuring. A prolapsed cord is not a painful complication but it is very frightening because of the danger to the baby. Do not leave the

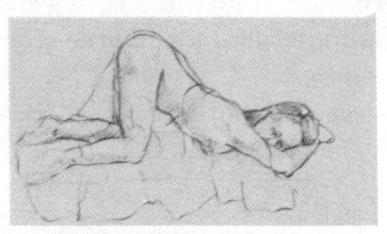

KNEE-CHEST POSITION

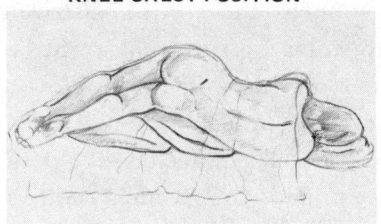

SIDE-LYING POSITION

If the cord can be seen, the expectant mother should be placed so the hips are elevated. If pillows are not immediately available, place her in knee-chest position temporarily. Then help her to turn on her side with pillows under her hips until medical help arrives.

mother unattended and tell her that all possible measures are being taken to bring about a safe delivery.

Protect the Cord

The cord is the baby's lifeline. If you feel that medical help cannot be obtained within a few minutes, very carefully wrap the cord — that is protruding beyond the vulva — in a warm, moist towel. Caution: Never try to place the cord back into the vagina. Do not press on the cord at any time.

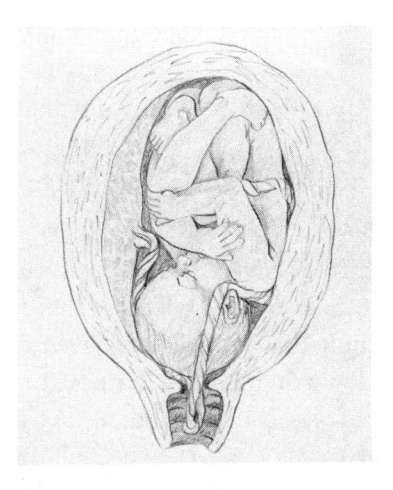

Fig. 8-10 If the umbilical cord emerges before the baby, the baby's life is in danger because the cord is squeezed between the baby and the mother's bony pelvis. Note that part of the cord is under the right shoulder, shutting off the blood supply.

MULTIPLE BIRTHS

When two or more embryos develop in the uterus at the same time, the expectant mother usually experiences greater discomforts and risks than the woman with a single pregnancy. A twin pregnancy is likely to cause more heaviness, lower abdominal pressure, and backache. Premature labors, toxemia, and hemorrhage are more common than with the woman who has one fetus in the uterus.

The expectant mother usually knows if she is carrying more than one baby. If this is not known, however, a multiple birth can be suspected when:

- the abdomen is unusually large before delivery
- the abdomen stays very large after the delivery of a baby

Multiple-birth deliveries usually occur quickly, with little help needed. This is due to the fact that multiple-birth babies are generally smaller than single-birth babies. Because of the small size, each fetus can move along the birth canal more easily.

Labor often begins for a multiple birth as much as two weeks earlier than anticipated for a single birth. Unless the woman is anticipating this fact, she may be unprepared when labor begins.

COMPLICATIONS AND UNUSUAL DELIVERIES 141

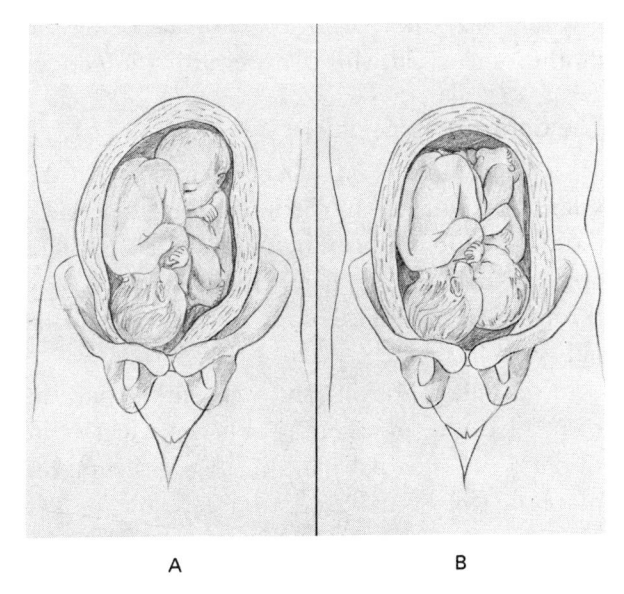

A   B

Fig. 8-11 Two positions assumed by twins. In (A) the first baby will deliver head first, the second by breech. In (B) each will deliver head first.

Labor And Delivery

Labor and delivery for a multiple birth should proceed much the same as for a single birth. After the first baby is born, contractions continue and the second baby is born — usually within a few minutes. The second baby is often in the breech position; this should not cause any complications, however, because of its smaller size. Emphasis should be directed toward (1) keeping the babies warm, (2) helping them breathe, (3) preventing hemorrhage in the mother and child, and (4) preventing infection.

The Cord and Placenta(s)

When a second birth is indicated, the umbilical cord of the first baby must be tied. **Caution:** Do not cut it. The cord is tied to prevent the second baby from hemorrhaging through the umbilical cord if there should be only one placenta.

A multiple-birth baby may either have its own placenta or share a placenta with the other(s). If each baby has its own placenta, the placenta will be expelled after each birth. The placentas should be tagged as number 1, number 2, etc. for the doctor's information when he examines the placentas. When there is only one placenta, it will deliver after the last baby. Expulsion may be more difficult because of its larger size.

Postdelivery Care

There is a greater tendency for the mother to hemorrhage after a multiple delivery. Care should be taken to be sure the mother's uterus remains firm after the delivery. It is essential to keep the babies warm after delivery because of their smaller size. Note: Since the babies are small, oxygen and resuscitation efforts are more likely to be needed.

THE STILLBORN

If the baby does not breathe at birth and does not respond to resuscitation efforts, it is said to be *stillborn*. If a baby is stillborn or appears to be dying shortly after delivery, it may console the parents to know that the baby has been baptized.

Anyone can baptize in an emergency situation regardless of his or her religious beliefs. However, the procedure must be done properly:

1. Sprinkle drops of water on the baby's forehead.
2. If the infant appears to be dying — while sprinkling the water say, "I baptize thee in the name of the Father, and of the Son, and of the Holy Spirit." Use these exact words. If the child appears to be dead — it should be baptized conditionally: while sprinkling the water, say "If there be life, I baptize thee in the name of the Father, and of the Son, and of the Holy Spirit."
3. Continue efforts to revive the baby during and following the baptism.

Give the mother the option of seeing and holding her stillborn infant. She will need as much emotional and psychological support as possible. The baby should be wrapped in a sheet, towel, or small blanket and transported to the hospital. Be sure it is identified with the name of the parents, sex of the child, place, date, and time of birth; and any additional comments which may be pertinent such as the baptism, first name — if it was expressed by the mother, etc.

MISCARRIAGE (ABORTION)

A spontaneous abortion is sometimes called a miscarriage by the public. However, abortion is the medical term used for all terminations of pregnancy before the fetus can live outside the mother's womb, regardless of whether or not the abortion is spontaneous or is induced. The fetus normally cannot survive if born before the sixth month of pregnancy. A spontaneous abortion (miscarriage) is often caused by a fall; also some women are simply unable to carry a fetus to term.

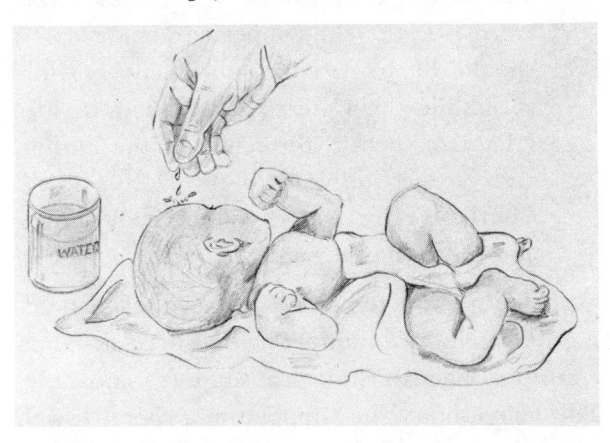

Fig. 8-12 "I baptize thee in the name of the Father, and of the Son, and of the Holy Spirit."

Excessive bleeding is the greatest danger. The bleeding may be internal or external; at times both may be present. If the bleeding is external, it can readily be seen. Signs and symptoms of internal bleeding are:
- Rapid, weak pulse
- Sudden drop in blood pressure
- Pallor of skin
- Cold, clammy skin
- Fainting or dizziness
- Sometimes vomiting of substance that looks like coffee grains (blood mixed with digested contents)

If internal bleeding is slow and lasts for several hours, patient shows apathy, lethargy, and confusion or restlessness. When an abortion occurs, control the bleeding, treat the woman for shock, and save the expelled fetus, membranes, and placenta.

Control Bleeding
- Place a sanitary napkin or clean cloth over the vaginal opening to absorb the blood. **Caution:** Never try to pack the vagina with absorbent materials.
- Send for medical help immediately.

Treat For Shock
- Treat the woman for shock by having her lie on her back with her legs and feet elevated.

- Cover the woman with a blanket, or whatever is available, in order to keep her warm.

Save Expelled Contents

- Save anything that is passed from the birth canal for the doctor to examine. **Caution:** Never try to replace or pull the fetus or umbilical cord out, if either is showing. Doing this could cause severe bleeding.
- As with the stillborn or dying newborn, baptize the fetus. Use the conditional form. While sprinkling water over it, say, "If there be life, I baptize thee in the name of the Father, and of the Son, and of the Holy Spirit."

SECTION 3
AFTER CHILDBIRTH

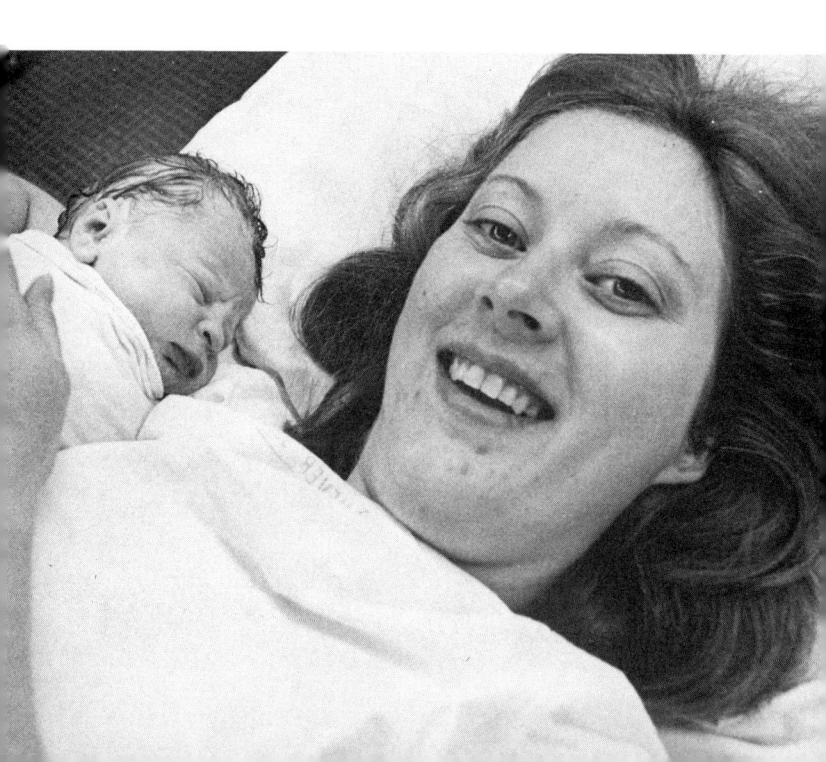

-9-
Postnatal Care of the Mother and New Baby

The first hour after delivery is vital to the well-being of the new mother. She should be closely observed for any adverse reactions. The fundus of her uterus should be checked frequently to be sure it remains firm and there is no excessive bleeding. If the fundus becomes limp, it must be massaged until it is again firm.

Care of the mother immediately after delivery, is directed to her comfort and safety.

1. Cleanse the vulva with a clean moist cloth. If available, warm soapy water may be poured over the vaginal opening. Pour the water from above towards the rectum. Rinse in the same manner with warm water.
2. If the perineum has been torn during delivery, treat it as an open wound by applying direct pressure to the bleeding area with a gauze pad or clean cloth. (If bleeding is severe, elevate the mother's hips and legs.)
3. Cover the vaginal opening with a sanitary napkin or clean cotton cloth. Apply the pad from front to back. A clean towel

may be placed under the buttocks for comfort and to catch any extra drainage.
4. Replace used sheets and blankets with clean dry ones.
5. Wipe the mother's face and hands with a damp cloth and dry with a clean towel in order to refresh her.
6. Keep the mother warm. Many women experience chilling after childbirth; an extra blanket and warm liquids may help to maintain the body's temperature.
7. Give the mother as much liquid as she desires, unless she is nauseous or for other reasons this is not advisable. The mother usually is very thirsty after delivery because of the loss of fluid during labor and delivery.
8. Transport to hospital as soon as possible.

Remember that the mother has just gone through a tremendous physical and emotional experience and will appreciate small acts of kindness. After she has delivered her baby, she may be exhausted and tense. Sleep may come easily after the delivery. On the other hand, she may be too excited about the childbirth experience. If she cannot sleep, encourage her to lie quietly and rest. Some women will have afterpains which are caused by the contractions of the uterus as it returns to its prepregnancy stage; this process is called involution. Also, there may be pain in the area of the perineum. Lying on her back may be helpful in relieving the discomfort.

Watch the general condition of the new mother. Whenever possible, blood flow, pulse, temperature, and blood pressure should be checked (every 15-20 minutes) for possible hemorrhage, shock, and infection. The fundus of the uterus should be checked for hardness and location.

- Vaginal drainage. If more than two sanitary napkins are saturated with bloody drainage during the first hour after delivery, there is excessive bleeding. The normal flow of vaginal blood within the first two hours after delivery is about two ounces. There should be no clots in the blood. If blood flow increases, the uterus should be massaged until it becomes firm.
- Pulse. After delivery, there may be a slight drop in the pulse rate; it may be 60 to 80 beats per minute. **Caution:** A fast pulse may be a sign of shock or concealed hemorrhage. Obtain medical help immediately.
- Temperature. Slight rises in temperature may occur following delivery. In general, the temperature should remain within normal limits.

- Blood Pressure. If equipment is available, the blood pressure should be taken and noted. It is not uncommon for a new mother to complain of a headache. Lying flat on her back may help to avoid the headache.
- Fundus. The top of the uterus should be hard and firm. It should be located below the navel (belly button). If the fundus is soft or large, massage gently with a circular motion until it is firm. Normally, the uterus will quickly respond to massage. Do not overmassage.

Keep a written record of these observations so that the physician may be informed of the progress and condition of the new mother.

THE NEW BABY

The healthy newborn has a lusty cry. When the baby cries, a deep flush spreads over its entire body. The skin may be covered with a white, cheesy protective coating called *vernix caseosa*. (There is no need to remove this after delivery.)

It is not necessary to clean the baby's skin or to wash its eyes, ears, or nose. This will be done when the baby is taken to the hospital. The baby should, however, be dried off and kept warm. The skin itself is thin and dry and veins may be seen through it. The skin on the baby's hands and feet is loose and wrinkled.

The normal newborn has a short neck, sloping shoulders, a large rounded abdomen and a narrow pelvis. It moves its arms and legs freely. The legs are often drawn up against the abdomen in the prenatal position. The baby's hands are clenched and flail the air.

The baby reacts to light by blinking, frowning, or closing its eyes. Since the baby cannot control eye movements, it may appear cross-eyed. The newborn reacts to loud or sudden sounds. It wakes and sleeps without any apparent pattern. It can taste and smell. It is sensitive to heat and cold. The newborn's body temperature by rectum is between 97° and 99° Fahrenheit (36° to 37° Celsius). The new baby sleeps about 16 to 20 hours a day, and awakes when hungry and uncomfortable.

The normal full-term baby has pudgy cheeks, a broad, flat nose, receding chin, and puffy eyelids. Birth weight ranges from 5 1/2 to 10 pounds. The average weight for boys is 7 1/2 pounds; girls weigh a little less. The overall length of the baby is about 18 to 21 inches (48-52 centimeters). The head seems large for its body. The bones in the head have not grown together and soft spots (fontanels) can be felt. One fontanel is located above the brow; the other is at the crown of the head, near the back.

The newborn baby looks surprisingly complete in contrast to its size. The hands resemble those of an adult with fingerprints, fingernails, and creases on the palms.

Body Support for the Newborn

While in the uterus, the infant did not have to support its own weight or maintain its own balance because the amniotic fluid provided a weightless environment. The amniotic sac offered little resistance to movements, yet gave the infant a sense of security by providing a point of contact whenever he reached out. After birth, when the baby reaches out and does not find a point of contact he may have a feeling of falling into space. This produces a reaction known as the Moro reflex. The *Moro reflex*, also known as the startle reflex, is a defensive response of newborns. The infant tenses, throws its arms out in an embracing motion and cries loudly. This can occur when the infant is asleep or awake.

At birth, the infant is still not able to support himself and must depend on others for comfort and support. The baby needs to find a point of contact whenever it reaches out in order to feel secure. The main purpose for providing support, however, is safety; the baby must be protected from injury.

Lifting the Baby

The newborn is very slippery and can be quite wriggly. Therefore, for safety reasons, it is best to have two points of contact when handling the new baby. In other words, *always* provide support to two parts of the body, usually the head and lower extremities.

Whenever a baby is carried or lifted, the head must be supported. It is larger and heavier than the rest of the body and the infant does not yet have control over its movements. **Caution:** Do not lift a baby by pulling on its arms. They are not strong enough to support the weight.

An infant lying on its back can be lifted easily and safely by the following method:

1. Face the baby's side.
2. Slide one hand under the head and neck and grasp the baby around the outer arm.
3. Support the baby's head with your forearm.
4. Slide your other hand under the baby's legs and grasp the feet while holding one finger between the ankles. (Instead of the feet, the thigh of the baby's outer leg could be grasped.)
5. Gently lift the baby.

Another method is to lift the baby while facing its feet.

1. Face the baby's feet.

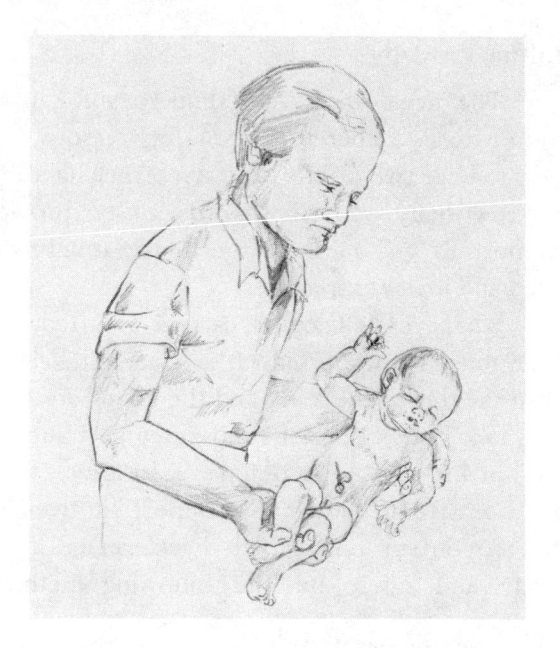

Fig. 9-1 A proper way to lift a newborn

2. Slightly lift baby's legs and buttocks by grasping his feet with one hand. Place a finger between his ankles to keep the ankles separated.
3. With palm up, slide the other hand under the full length of the baby until the entire back and head are supported.
4. Gently lift the baby.

Other methods of lifting and supporting the newborn are described and illustrated in the Appendix.

-10-
Arriving at the Hospital

The emergency medical technician, law enforcement officer, ambulance team member, or other person accompanying the woman in labor should have information available for the admitting clerk and nurse on duty in the labor and delivery room of the hospital. Some general facts are obtained whether the woman is in labor or has delivered. In addition, specific information is necessary according to whether the woman is in labor or has delivered.

In all cases, the name, address, telephone number of the expectant mother and the nearest living relative (parents, child's father) must be obtained. It is also necessary for the hospital personnel to know the religion of the expectant mother and whether the woman has delivered or is still undelivered. The name of the doctor is also necessary. These general facts should be obtained on all expectant and childbirth cases.

It is also helpful to know: whether this is the first pregnancy, the estimated due date, whether or not prenatal care has been given, and

158 AFTER CHILDBIRTH

UPON ADMISSION

- Mother's name, address, and phone number
- Name, address, and phone number of nearest living relative (parents, father of child)
- Mother's religion
- Condition of the mother — delivered, undelivered
- Number of this pregnancy — include miscarriages
- How many past deliveries (number of live births)
- Estimated due date
- Doctor's name
- Has prenatal care been given?
- Blood type (if known)

Fig. 10-1 Facts usually required for hospitalization of a maternity patient (also see figure 10-2 or 10-3).

the blood type of the parents. If this is not the first pregnancy, how many children has she had? Figure 10-1 summarizes what basic information must be obtained in all cases. Additional facts are to be obtained — depending on whether the baby has been born or not. These are described in figures 10-2 and 10-3.

If Delivery HAS Taken Place —
- Place and time of delivery
- Sex of child
- Pulse and respirations (blood pressure, if known)
- Amount of bleeding (loss of blood and present status)
- Condition of the fundus: is it firm or soft?
- Time placenta was delivered
- Condition of baby and mother

Fig. 10-2 Additional information required (see figure 10-1)

If Delivery Has NOT Taken Place —
- When did contractions start
- Length and strength of contraction (duration, intensity)
- Length of time between contractions (frequency)
- Pulse and respirations (blood pressure, if known)
- Last time medication and/or food was consumed
- Has the bag of waters ruptured; if so, at what time
- Is there a bloody show; if so, when was it first noticed
- Is there meconium present; if so, when was it first noticed

Fig. 10-3 Additional information required (see figure 10-1)

SECTION 4
APPENDIX

A-1 List of Emergency Supplies
A-2 Lamaze Techniques
A-3 Ways to Hold an Infant
A-4 Terms Related to Childbirth
A-5 Optional Self Test and Answers

EMERGENCY CHILDBIRTH SUPPLIES

4 clean towels

2 folded sheets

1 receiving blanket for the baby

Gauze squares

Small rubber bulb (ear) syringe

Alcohol

Sterilized scissors

Sterilized ties or clamps
(for umbilical cord)

Diapers

Safety pins

Basin or pan
(in case mother vomits)

Blanket for mother

Pillow for mother

Sanitary napkins

Plastic bag or container
(for the afterbirth)

Newspapers or plastic bags
(to protect car upholstery)

Flashlight
(if trip is at night)

Fig. A-1 A list of supplies to be taken along when transporting a laboring woman to medical care. These can be used in the event the birth occurs en route.

A-2
Lamaze Techniques

A natural childbirth method, called *psychoprophylaxis*, has become very popular in recent years. Dr. Fernand Lamaze of Paris brought this technique to Western Europe in 1952. It is considered superior to earlier methods. Psychoprophylaxis depends upon educating the mother-to-be about childbirth and training her — by exercise and breathing techniques — to control her activity during labor. It is an intellectual, physical, and emotional preparation for childbirth.

Childbirth, no matter how normal, is accompanied by some degree of discomfort. Exercise using the psychoprophylactic method is based on what is known as the theory of conditioned reflexes. It takes advantage of the fact that the brain can accept only one set of signals at a time. If the stronger set is one of conditioned response to exercise and control of the body muscles to expel the baby, instead of one of unpleasant pain, then it takes precedence over the signal from the uterine contractions.

The use of Lamaze techniques can help maintain relaxation during labor. By concentrating on techniques, the awareness of pain during contractions can be greatly reduced.

The Lamaze method of pain control includes physical relaxation, the sense of sight (focal point), the sense of touch (effleurage) and specific breathing patterns.

PHYSICAL RELAXATION

Physical relaxation enables the uterus to work more efficiently and reduces the degree of fatigue and tension. To teach the mother to relax, give the following instructions:

1. Sigh repeatedly. As the air goes out, let specific parts of the body collapse, such as the toes, the foot, the legs, the knees, the thighs, the abdomen, the fingers, the wrist, the left arm, the right arm, etc.
2. Imagine you are floating or you are very, very heavy; or you are disappearing or growing smaller.
3. Count backwards from 100 until you are completely relaxed; work toward complete relaxation as soon as you begin the countdown.

When labor begins, total concentration should be applied to relaxation. When relaxation techniques are not enough to control discomfort, the first level of breathing should be started.

FOCAL POINT

There is a tendency to become more aware of pain when isolated by closing the eyes; therefore, the Lamaze technique is done with the eyes open. The mother should choose a point on which to focus and keep her eyes fixed on that point throughout the contraction.

EFFLEURAGE

Effleurage is a light massage that can be soothing and can help in relaxation when it is done by the woman herself or by someone else. It can be given when the expectant mother is in either a sitting or lying position.

- *Sitting position*: Place the hands over the pubic area. Slowly and firmly bring each hand (right hand around right side, left hand around left side) around the sides of the uterus, over the fundus, and down midline to your starting position (an outline similar to butterfly wings).
- *Left side-lying position*: Place the right hand close to the left hip bone. Gently and firmly sweep your hand down towards the pubic bone and up towards the right hip. Return hand to its starting position. This massage can also be done by someone other than the mother. The person would sit or stand facing the mother's back and reach over to begin at the left hip.

These movements are most effective when done rhythmically and gently enough to avoid irritation and yet firmly enough to avoid tickling. They are easier to do and are more effective over bare skin. Cornstarch on the hands will help keep effleurage smooth. Although effleurage can be used throughout labor, it is not uncommon for some women to be irritated by touch during intense contractions.

BREATHING PATTERNS

There are three levels of breathing patterns: deep chest, accelerated, and transition. All are done with the chest to avoid pressure on the contracting uterus. An organizing breath is taken at the beginning of each contraction and a relaxing breath at the end. The *organizing breath* is a deep, lateral chest breath used to prepare the woman for the contraction; the *relaxing breath* is a deep, lateral chest breath used to help release any tension built up during the contraction. The woman should breathe in through the nose and out through the mouth.

Deep Chest Breathing

1. Contraction begins.
2. Take an organizing breath.
3. While the contraction is lasting, breathe in through the nose; breathe out through the

mouth. Take 6 to 10 breaths per minute. Keep shoulders and abdomen relaxed. Be aware of the outgoing breath passing over the lips.
4. Contraction ends.
5. Take a deep relaxing breath and completely relax.

Observations. Change from deep chest breathing to accelerated breathing when there is:

- Increased respiratory rate (beyond 18 breaths a minute)
- Difficulty in attempts to slow down the rate of breathing
- Increased tension and difficulty in relaxing at the peak of contraction
- Restlessness throughout the contractions

Accelerated Breathing

1. Contraction begins.
2. Take an organizing breath — quicker one now, but still deep.
3. Breathe in through nose and out through mouth — as in deep chest breathing.
4. As contraction increases in intensity and reaches its peak, breathe faster to keep ahead of contraction. At this time breaths are in and out through the mouth at a rate of about one per second. This is shallow breathing with maximum movement in the

upper chest. Note: Remember that air exchange must be equal to prevent hyperventilation.
5. Slow down as contraction decreases in intensity.
6. Contraction ends.
7. Take a deep relaxing breath and completely relax.

Observations. Signs to look for in deciding to change from accelerated breathing to transition breathing are:

- Spontaneous increase in rate of breathing
- Inability to stay relaxed through the contraction even with accelerated breathing
- The urge to push or bear down at the peak of a contraction

The woman should try to breathe at the slowest rate as long as possible. The slower rates are usually less tiring. Transition begins when the cervix is 7-8 cm dilated and ends with full dilatation (10 cm). It is the shortest but most intense phase of the first stage of labor.

Transition Breathing

1. Contraction begins.
2. Take an organizing breath — contractions are beginning to peak sooner so this breath may need to be quicker (shorter) than before.

3. Begin breathing in and out through the mouth at about one breath per second.
4. Every 4th, 5th or 6th expiration blow out gently with a "puh" sound. Become comfortable with your own rate and stay consistent. Count to self, "one, two, three, four, puh," etc.
5. Contraction ends.
6. Take a deep relaxing breath and completely relax.
7. Prepare to begin again.

Controlling the Urge to Push. If a strong urge to push or bear down is felt and the cervix is not yet fully dilated, tip the chin back and use the "puh, puh, puh" breaths (of the transition breathing pattern) until the urge subsides. The times a woman in labor should **not** push are:

- Cervix is not fully dilated (first stage of labor)
- Crowning (bulging due to pressure of head against vaginal opening)

Also, if no one is in attendance to help with the delivery of the baby, the expectant mother should not attempt to hasten the delivery by pushing.

Pushing. The expectant mother should be encouraged to push during the second stage of labor. This is the period of time after the cervix has fully dilated and up to crowning. You will recall that crowning takes place towards the end of the second stage. **Caution:** No pushing is done during crowning. Have the expectant mother take light and rapid breaths (panting) to prevent pushing so the baby is allowed to pass gently through the vaginal opening. The times a laboring woman **should** push are:

- After cervix is fully dilated
- Before crowning takes place
- When the placenta is being expelled

Knowing the most effective way to push saves energy that might otherwise be wasted.

1. Contraction begins.
2. Take 3 quick deep breaths. On the third breath hold all the air in. Bring chin down to chest. Contract the abdominal muscles. Let the legs, especially the inner thighs, totally relax. Continue bearing down until most of the air is expelled from the lungs. Then very quickly let air out and take in more and continue bearing down until the contraction ends.
3. Relax until contraction begins again.

COACHING THE WOMAN IN LABOR

To help an expectant mother during labor, be prepared to:

1. Learn to look for periods of relaxation.

2. Coach breathing by verbal command or demonstration.
3. Know the progress of labor and delivery.
4. Recognize the signs that labor has begun.

If the membranes rupture or start to leak, note the time, amount (trickle or gush) and color. If the doctor — or hospital — has not been contacted, do so at once and take the expectant mother to the hospital.

Time the contractions and the intervals.

1. Time from the beginning of one contraction to the beginning of another one to determine whether they are getting longer, stronger, and closer together.
   a. Time the number of seconds that the contraction lasts.
   b. Time the period of relaxation (interval).
2. Place your hand on the abdomen over the uterus to feel the actual contractions from time to time to see how hard they are.
3. Remind the woman to breathe and relax with the contractions. When she can no longer walk or talk through a contraction, suggest she begin slow chest breathing.

Keep her relaxed and stay relaxed yourself.

1. Periodically remind her to keep her eyes open and be aware of the beginning and the end of the contractions.

2. Adjust physical environment for comfort, giving thought to light, noise, pillows, etc.
3. Encourage, praise, and reassure her.
4. Gently massage or apply pressure to the small of the back for backache.
5. Do not hold her hand during contractions. Remind her to leave her whole body, hands, feet, back of the neck, and lower jaw limp. Sigh deeply with her — relaxing is contagious.
6. Offer physical comforts such as a back rub, ice chips, or wet sponge for dryness of mouth.
7. After timing the contractions, inform the expectant mother so that she can time her breathing with the contractions.

If she has difficulty keeping in control she will probably:

1. Be unable to relax and may grip your hand or the bedsheet.
2. Be unable to continue breathing or keep a focal point throughout the entire contraction.
3. Be unable to be still during the contraction.

To help her gain control:

1. Help her resume her breathing by giving her firm confident commands to look at your

face and do what you do. Then you breathe while she imitates.
2. Massage her back or offer effleurage if it is helpful.
3. Between contractions, encourage her, and remind her what to do during the next contraction.

The transition stage begins when the cervix has dilated to about 3 to 3 1/2 inches (7-8 cm). Symptoms of the transition phase are:

- Increased low back pressure
- Vagueness, drowsiness, easily distracted, forgetful
- Irregular contractions: 1 to 3 minutes apart, lasting longer than before
- Feeling of pressure on the rectum
- Irritability
- Nausea or vomiting
- Shivering
- Hiccups or belching
- Urge to push or bear down
- Feelings of despair

Support during transition phase.

1. Encourage her; this is important to a woman in transition. Tell her how well she is doing and that it will soon be over.
2. Since it is so difficult to relax completely at this time, do your best to keep her engrossed with her breathing.

3. Remember how to do transition breathing. Do it with her.
4. Bathe her brow and neck with cool water.
5. Be prepared to give counter pressure on her lower back if she is having backache.
6. Be tactful in suggesting any change in her actions. Keep her informed of her labor progress.
7. Make her aware of your presence and your concern and support. Don't leave her alone at any time. Transition is the shortest but the most intense time of labor.

Pushing.

1. Help her find a comfortable position for pushing (usually a semireclined position, on her back, with knees bent and apart, feet on bed).
2. When a contraction begins, give her commands: Quickly breathe in, breathe out; breathe in, breathe out; breathe in, hold it, and bear down. Relaxing breath, relax and breathe normally after contraction ends.
3. Remind her to keep her mouth relaxed while pushing.
4. Give encouragement mixed with firm commands.

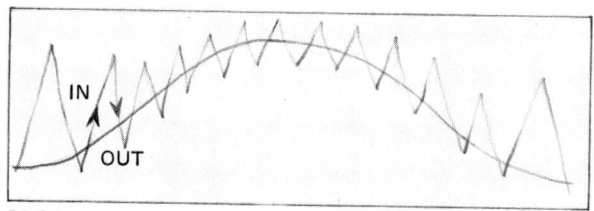

LAMAZE 175

DEEP CHEST PATTERN — 60 SECONDS 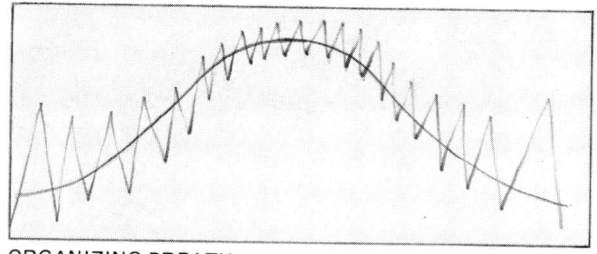
ORGANIZING BREATH · RELAXING BREATH

ACCELERATED PATTERN — 60 SECONDS 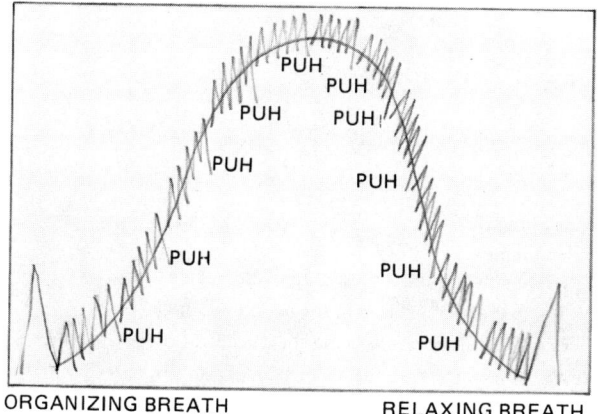
ORGANIZING BREATH · RELAXING BREATH

TRANSITION PATTERN — 60-75 SECONDS
ORGANIZING BREATH · RELAXING BREATH

Fig. A-2 Three breathing patterns

1. Contraction begins.
2. Take an organizing breath.
3. Begin pattern of breathing.
4. Concentrate on relaxation techniques.
5. Maintain a focal point throughout the contraction.
6. Effleurage
7. Continue breathing technique while maintaining focal point and concentrating on relaxation.
8. Contraction over
9. Take a relaxing breath.
10. Relax and rest (between contractions).
11. Repeat the process, beginning with next contraction.

The Lamaze Method

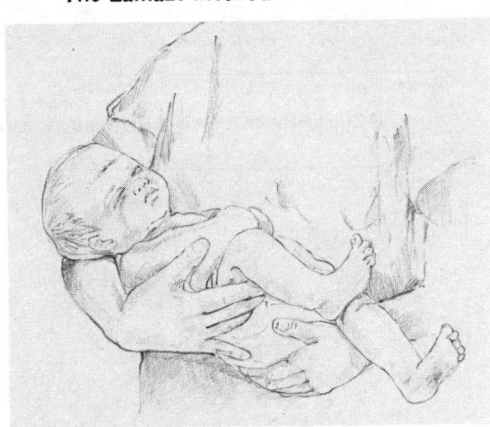

CRADLE HOLD

The cradle hold is one of the most common ways of holding an infant. A variation of it is usually used when feeding the baby.

1. Cradle the infant's head in the bend of your elbow.
2. Extend your forearm around the outside of the infant's body.
3. With the fingers of the same hand, grasp the outer leg.
4. Place your other hand on the infant's buttocks for additional support.

A-3 Ways to hold an infant (continued)

SHOULDER HOLD

The shoulder hold requires two hands to properly support the baby's back. This hold can be used when burping the baby.

1. Place the infant in an upright position with its arms and legs against your chest.
2. Rest the infant's head against your shoulder.
3. Support the infant's back with your forearm, and its head with your hand.
4. Support the baby's buttocks with the palm of your other hand.

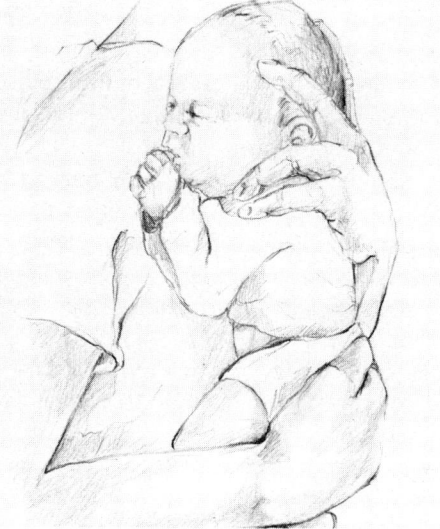

FOOTBALL HOLD

The football hold is a firm, secure hold that leaves one hand free to perform other duties. It is often used for rinsing the baby's head when giving it a bath.

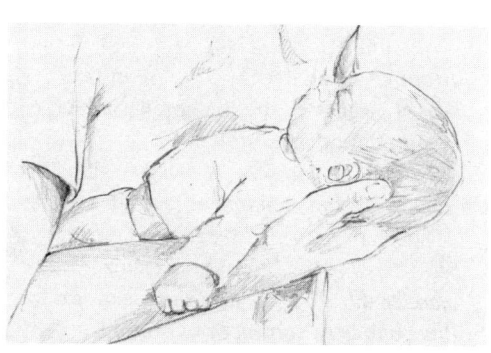

1. Place the baby's buttocks firmly between your hip and your elbow.
2. Support the baby's back with your forearm.
3. Support the baby's neck and head with your open hand.

A-3 Ways to hold an infant

A-4
TERMS RELATED TO CHILDBIRTH:
Pronunciation and Definition

abortion (ah-bor'shun) — termination of pregnancy before the fetus is capable of living outside the uterus

amenorrhea (ah-men"or-rhe'ah) — the absence or suppression of menstruation

amnion (am'nee-on) — a thin, transparent sac which holds the fetus suspended in amniotic fluid during gestation; also called the bag of waters

amniotic fluid (am-nee-ot'ik) — the transparent, slightly alkaline liquid surrounding the fetus within the amniotic sac

anal sphincter (ay'nal sfink'ter) — circular muscle which controls the passage of feces and flatus from the rectum

android pelvis (an'droyd) — angular wedge-shaped pelvis

anovulatory (an-oh'vu-la-to"ree) — menstruation without the discharge of an ovum

anterior (an-te'ree-or) — located before or toward the front

anus (ay'nus) — pigmented, puckered opening of the rectum

atrophy (at'row-fee) — decrease in size

bag of waters — the membranes which enclose the amniotic fluid; the amnion

Bartholin's gland (Bar'to-lins) — gland located on each side of the labia minora that secretes a lubricating substance during sexual intercourse

birth canal — the uterus and vagina

bladder (blad'der) — storage space for urine

Braxton-Hicks contractions — painless contractions of the uterus that occur periodically throughout pregnancy

breech — presentation of the buttocks, the hind part of the body

buttocks (but'tucks) — the fleshy, rounded lower part of the back, on which a person sits

cervix (ser'viks) — the neck or lower narrow end of the uterus

chorion (ko'ree-on) — outer layer of cells of the fertilized ovum which protects and nourishes it

chorionic villi (ko'ree-on'ik vil'eye) — vascular projections from the chorion

chromosome (kro'mo-sohm) — microscopic body that develops from the nucleus of a cell and contains the genes

cilia (sill'ee-ah) — hairlike projections that create a waving action in order to provide locomotion for something

circumcision (sir'kum-si'shun) — surgical removal of the foreskin of the penis

cleavage (klee'vej) — cell division which follows the fertilization of the ovum

clitoris (klit'or-is) — small, elongated mass of muscle and tissue located at the front of the vulva; it is extremely sensitive and responds to sexual excitation

coccyx (cock'sicks) — small, triangular bone found at the base of the spine

congenital (kon-jen'i-tal) — existing at birth

copulation (kop"u-lay'shun) — sexual intercourse

corpus luteum (kor'pus lu-tee'um) — the yellow mass of tissue formed from the ruptured graafian follicle; it secretes the hormone, progesterone

crowning — stage in delivery when the head of the fetus bulges at the vaginal opening

dartos (dar'tos) — contractile muscle fibers located within the scrotum

descent — continuous progress of the fetus as it passes through the birth canal

dilatation (dil"uh-tay'shun) — condition of being expanded beyond normal size *dystocia* (dis-toe' shah) — difficult labor

dysmenorrhea (dis-men"or-rhe'ah) — painful menstruation

effleurage (ef-flur-ahzh') — in massage, a deep or gentle stroking

ejaculation (ee-jak"u-lay'shun) — expulsion of semen from the penis

embryo (em'bree-oh) — term for the fertilized ovum between the second and eighth week after conception

endometrium (en"doh-mee'tree-um) — mucous membrane lining the inner surface of the uterus

engagement — when the presenting part of the fetus descends and fully enters the pelvis

epididymis (ep"ee-did'ee-mis) — small, oblong body resting upon and beside the posterior surface of the testis consisting of a long coiled tube; it is the principal storehouse for sperm

epithelium (ep"ee-thee'lee-um) — a layer of cells forming the surface layer of mucous membrane of the fallopian tubes and uterus

estrogen (es'tro-jen) — a female sex hormone produced by the ovaries

extension — unflexing of the baby's head as it pushes upward out of the vaginal canal

fallopian tubes (fah-lo'pee-an) — canals extending from the upper corners of the uterus to the abdominal cavity which carry the ovum from the ovary to the uterus

fertilization (fer"ti-li-zay'shun) — conception; sperm cell unites with the ovum through intercourse

fetus (fee'tus) — the fertilized ovum from the eighth week of gestation until birth

flexion (flek'shun) — the process of the fetal head being bent forward so that its chin rests on its breastbone in order for the narrowest part of the head to enter the pelvic outlet

TERMS 181

follicle (fol'lee-cle) — microscopic structure embedded in the connective tissues within the ovaries; each follicle contains an ovum and cells

fraternal twins — result when two ova are fertilized by two sperm cells; there are two amniotic sacs and separate or fused placentas

fundus (fun'dus) — the upper rounded part of the uterus

gene (jeen) — hereditary factor found in the chromosomes

genetics (jen-et'iks) — the study of heredity and its variations

gestation (jes-tay'shun) — period of development from conception to birth

glans penis (glanz pee'nis) — slightly enlarged structure at the end of the penis where the opening of the urethra is located

graafian follicle (graf'ee-an fol'lee-cle) — microscopic sac within the ovary, developed from a follicle, in which the ovum develops

gynecoid pelvis (guy'-nee-coy-d) — female, heart-shaped pelvis

hemorrhage (hem'er-raj) — profuse discharge of blood

hyaluronidase (hi-allure-on'-id-ace) — a cell dissolving enzyme

hydramnios (high-dram'nee-os) — overdistention of the uterus caused by too much amniotic fluid

hymen (high'men) — fold of mucous membrane partly closing the vaginal opening

identical twins — result from the union of one sperm cell and one ovum; there is one placenta and two amniotic sacs

impotent (im'poh-tent) — inability of the male to have an erection or ejaculation

interval — period between contractions

intrauterine (in"tra-u'ter-een) — within the uterus

in utero (in u'ter-oh) — within the uterus

182 TERMS

lanugo (la-noo'go) — fine downy hair covering the body of the fetus

lightening — the decreased abdominal distention felt when the uterus descends into the pelvic cavity; it usually occurs 2 to 3 weeks before the onset of labor

meconium (mek-ko'nee-um) — dark green substance consisting of bile, mucus, and cells which make up the newborn's first bowel movement

menarche (men-ar'kee) — the onset of menstrual function

menopause (men'oh-pawz) — the period which marks the permanent cessation of the menstrual function

menorrhagia (men-or-rah'jee-ah) — prolonged or excessive bleeding during the menstrual period

menstruation (men"stru-ay'shun) — the process of casting off the unnecessary uterine lining when conception does not occur

metrorrhagia (met-roh-rah'jee-ah) — bleeding from the uterus at a time other than the menstrual period

mons veneris (mons ven'er-is) — pad of fat covering the pubic area

multipara (mul-tip'ah-rah) — a woman who has borne more than one child

ovaries (oh'var-eez) — the sex glands of the female which mature and discharge the ova and produce hormones necessary to the process of reproduction; they are almond-shaped bodies lying on either side of the pelvic cavity

ovulation (oh'vu-lay-shun) — the process by which a mature ovum is released and the uterus is made ready to receive the fertilized ovum

ovum (oh'vum) — the female reproductive cell

oxytocin (ock"see-toh'sin) — hormone secreted by the pituitary gland that causes the uterus to contract

pelvis — bony structure that makes up the hips; contains 5 bones and is part and extension of lower spine *penis* (pee'nis) — the male organ of copulation which also contains the passage for urine

perineum (per"ee-nee'um) — the external area between the vagina and the anus in the female; between the scrotum and anus in a male

peritoneum (per"ee-toh-nee'um) — a transparent membrane that lines the abdominal cavity

pituitary gland (peh-tew'eh-terr"ee) — a small, gray, rounded body attached to the base of the brain which produces various internal secretions directly or indirectly affecting most basic body functions.

placenta (plah-sen'tah) — a spongy, oval structure in the uterus that provides oxygen and nourishment to the fetus and discharges fetal waste products; it is developed from the outer rim of the fertilized ovum and the uterine lining where the ovum is embedded. When expelled after birth, it is known as the afterbirth.

position — term used to designate the part of the fetus in relation to the mother's pelvis

posterior — situated toward the back; coming after

prepuce (pree'poos) — fold of skin covering the glans penis in the male; the foreskin

presentation (pree"zen-tay'shun) — term used to designate the part of the fetus that is nearest the opening of the vagina

primipara (pry-mip'ah-rah) — a woman who is giving birth to her first child

progesterone (proh-jes'tur-ohn) — a hormone produced in the corpus luteum that prepares the uterine lining for the reception and development of the fertilized ovum

prolapsed cord (proh-laps'ed) — the protrusion of the umbilical cord from the vagina before the birth of the fetus *prostate gland* (pros'tate) — gland in the male that surrounds the neck of the bladder and the urethra; it secretes a milky substance into the semen which neutralizes the acidic fluid from the testes, thereby stimulating the sperm to action

puberty (pew'ber-tee) — age when the reproductive organs become functional, usually between the 11th and 16th year of life

pubis (pew'bis) — the bone forming the front of the pelvis

quickening (kwik'en-ing) — first movements of the fetus which can be felt

rectum (reck'tum) — terminal portion of the large intestine

sacrum (say'krum) — large wedge-shaped bone which forms the posterior wall of the pelvis

scrotum (skroh'tum) — pouch of loose skin that contains the testes in the male

semen (see'men) — fluid which carries the sperm cells

seminal vesicle glands (sem'eh-nal ves'eh-cle) — two saclike structures lying behind the bladder in the male; they secrete a fluid which is part of the semen

show — vaginal discharge consisting of thick, stringy mucus streaked with blood that is discharged from the vagina before or during labor

spermatozoa (spur"muh-toh-zoh'ah) — the male reproductive cells

sternum (stur'num) — flat narrow bone in midline of the chest

testes (tes'tees) — the primary sex organs of the male; they produce sperm and the male sex hormone

testosterone (tes-tos'teer-ohn) — the male sex hormone

transition phase — period just before expulsion (second stage of labor)

umbilical cord (um-bill'ikal) — the attachment that connects the fetus with the placenta *ureters* (u'reh-ters) — the tubes that carry urine from the kidneys to the bladder

urethra (u-ree'thra) — a tube used to discharge urine from the bladder

urinary meatus (u'reh-nar'ee mee-ay'tus) — opening located below the clitoris through which urine is discharged

uterus (u'ter-us) — muscular, pear-shaped female organ where fertilized ovum is nourished and grown

vagina (vah-ji'nah) — tubelike passage leading from the vulva to the uterus; it is located between the urethra and the rectum

vas deferens (vas def'er-enz) — a slim muscular tube which carries the sperm from the testes to the urethra

vasectomy (vas-ek'toh-mee) — surgical operation to prevent the sperm from traveling beyond the vas deferens

vernix caseosa (ver'niks kay"see-oh'sah) — cheeselike substance covering the fetus

vulva (vuhl'vah) — external parts of the female genital organs, lying beneath the mons veneris

zygote (zy'goat) — the fertilized egg cell

Positions Assumed by Expectant Mother During Pregnancy and/or Labor (Drape with sheet)

Dorsal Recumbent — Flat on back. Knees flexed. Legs slightly separated with feet flat on bed. Pillow under head.

Lithotomy — Like dorsal recumbent except that both feet are placed in stirrups so that knees are flexed and separated.

Sims' — Lie on left side with small pillow under head. Left arm placed behind body. Right arm up front. Left leg slightly bent while right leg is flexed on abdomen, resting on a pillow.

Modified Sims' — Sidelying position with pillows under hips; used for prolapse of cord.

Knee-Chest — On abdomen. Head on small pillow and turned to one side. Knees on bed but flexed and drawn up toward chest. Difficult position to maintain. Never leave alone. Used for pelvic exams and when prolapse of cord occurs.

Semi-Fowler's — Resting position. On back. Head and shoulders elevated to 45 degree angle. Knees slightly flexed. Heels on bed.

A-5
SELF TEST

1. Name the 3 stages of labor.
2. Explain the difference between true and false labor pains.
3. What is the "show"? How does it differ from the fluid from the rupture of the bag of waters?
4. What is the usual length of time a woman is in labor if she is having her first baby?
5. Name 4 signs that indicate labor is not progressing normally.
6. When evaluating the state of the woman in labor, what three questions should you ask the woman regarding her labor?
7. Name 5 signs that indicate delivery is imminent.
8. Describe how to prepare the woman when an emergency delivery is about to take place.
9. Why is it important to take time to properly drape the woman when an emergency birth is occurring?
10. When should the expectant mother *not* bear down with her contractions?
11. What should you tell the woman to do when the baby's head starts to emerge?

188 SELF TEST

12. What should be done if the umbilical cord is wrapped around the baby's neck?

13. After the head is delivered, how can you assist the delivery of the shoulders, if they do not deliver after two contractions?

14. Describe the immediate care of the newborn.

15. What steps can be taken if, after clearing the mucus from the baby, the baby still does not breathe?

16. Explain how to give mouth-to-mouth resuscitation to the newborn.

17. Explain cardiopulmonary resuscitation of the newborn.

18. Why is it essential to squeeze the air from the bulb when using a bulb syringe to suction *before* inserting the syringe into the baby's mouth or nose?

19. Explain how to properly massage the woman's uterus after the baby has been born.

20. Name 3 signs that indicate the placenta has separated from the wall of the uterus.

21. After delivery of the placenta, how should the uterus feel? What should be done if it does not feel this way?

22. Why must the uterus be firm before the placenta is delivered?

SELF TEST 189

23. Name 5 things that should be done if the woman is hemorrhaging.

24. Describe how to properly cut the umbilical cord.

25. If there is bleeding from the umbilical cord after it has been tied and cut, what should you do?

26. What should you do if the part presenting at the vaginal opening is not the baby's head or buttocks?

27. What should be done if contractions are 2 minutes apart and birth is not occurring within 20 minutes?

28. What do you do if the baby's head does not deliver within 3 minutes after the body when the birth is a breech delivery?

29. In what position do you immediately place the woman if a prolapsed cord is discovered?

30. If the baby is premature, what precautions do you need to take in giving it care?

31. What may alert you to the fact that a multiple birth should be expected, if this information is not known?

32. When the emergency delivery is a multiple birth, what three complications are more likely to occur?

33. Describe the immediate care of the mother after delivery.

34. Explain why the baby's head should be supported whenever it is lifted or carried.

35. Name 5 signs of internal bleeding.

36. What should be done if the baby is stillborn?

ANSWERS TO SELF TEST

1. The three stages of labor are the dilatation stage, the expulsion stage, and the placental stage.

2. True labor pains recur with rhythmic regularity and gradually increase in frequency, intensity, and duration. They usually radiate from the back to the front of the abdomen. Contractions are accompanied by abdominal tightening, pain or discomfort, and rarely exceed 60 seconds. They are not relieved by the woman's activity. The contractions shorten the cervix and widen its opening; the "show" is present. False labor pains are not always painful and may last from 3 to 4 minutes. They are irregular in frequency, intensity, and duration. They are usually confined to the lower abdomen. False labor pains are relieved by a warm bath or slight activity such as walking. The cervix does not shorten or widen with the pains; no "show" is present.

3. The "show" is a vaginal discharge consisting of thick, stringy mucus streaked with blood. The fluid from the rupture of the bag of waters is a colorless water-type fluid.

4. The usual length of time a woman is in labor for her first baby is 12 to 15 hours.

5. Signs that indicate labor is not progressing normally are:
   - Abnormal vaginal bleeding.
   - Contractions stop after labor has begun.
   - A rise in blood pressure.
   - A rigid uterus after a contraction is over.
   - Severe headache and dizziness.
   - Passage of meconium-stained fluid (unless baby is in breech position)
   - Umbilical cord can be seen at vagina.

6. Three questions to ask a woman in labor when evaluating her state are: (1) How long has she been in labor, (2) Is this her first baby, (3) What is the length of time between contractions.

7. Five signs that indicate delivery is imminent are:
   - Time from the beginning of one contraction to the beginning of the next contraction is approximately two minutes or less.
   - The woman is straining or pushing down with the contractions.
   - The woman feels she must move her bowels.
   - The woman is crying out warning the baby is coming.
   - The baby's head can be seen at the vaginal opening at the time of contractions.

8. In order to prepare the woman for an emergency delivery, explain to her what you are going to do before you do it. If the birth is occurring in a public place, provide as much privacy as possible by shielding the scene from the view of others. Have the woman remove her clothing from the lower half of her body and lie on a firm surface with her knees bent and her legs spread apart. Be sure her head is elevated. Place clean towels, folded linen, newspapers, or clothing under her buttocks. Place a clean towel or sheet on the woman's abdomen. Cover each thigh with a clean towel or sheet (or whatever is available). Only the vaginal opening should be exposed.

9. Draping the woman is important because it saves unnecessary embarrassment and will help her be more relaxed; it also provides a sanitary environment.

10. The laboring woman should not bear down with her contractions when the baby's head starts to emerge, or when she is not fully dilated.

11. When the baby's head starts to emerge, tell the woman to stop pushing. Ask her to pant or take frequent short breaths, puff out her cheeks and blow the air out through pursed lips.

194 ANSWERS

12. If the umbilical cord is wrapped around the baby's neck, carefully and quickly loosen the cord with your forefinger placed between the cord and the baby's neck. If the cord is loose enough, slip it over the baby's head. If the cord is too tight and cannot be loosened, it must be clamped or tied off in two places and cut immediately.

13. If the shoulders do not deliver after two contractions from the time the head is delivered, apply a gentle but firm downward pressure on the baby's head to help deliver the upper shoulder. Gently raise the baby's head to deliver the lower shoulder.

14. Grasp the baby's ankles firmly with one hand as the feet are born. Support the head with the other hand while you raise the baby's legs. (This helps the mucus to drain.) Dry the baby with a towel and place it head down on its side between the mother's legs. Wipe away remaining mucus. With your hand, gently stroke the baby's chest upward towards its mouth. Wipe the mucus from the baby's mouth again. Suction the baby's mouth and nose with a bulb syringe, if available, to remove mucus. Check the heart rate. If it is much lower than 100 beats per minute, vigorously massage the baby with a dry towel to stimulate it.

Cover the baby with a towel or blanket to keep it warm. Remember to handle the baby gently, keep it warm, and avoid contaminating it as much as possible.

15. After clearing the mouth and nose of mucus, if the baby still does not breathe:
    - Rub the baby's back or chest briskly but gently.
    - If no response after 30 seconds, hold the baby's ankles together with one hand. With the forefingers of the other hand, snap sharply against the soles of the baby's feet. Repeat after 30 seconds if there is no response.
    - If there is still no response, do mouth-to-mouth resuscitation.
    - If there is no response from mouth-to-mouth resuscitation and you cannot locate a pulse after 2 minutes, begin cardiopulmonary resuscitation.

16. In order to give mouth-to-mouth resuscitation to the newborn:
    - Clear the baby's mouth of any mucus.
    - Place your hand at the base of the baby's neck to tilt its head back slightly.
    - Place your mouth over the baby's nose and mouth creating a tight seal.

- Gently blow small puffs of air from your cheeks into the baby's nose and mouth (about one puff every 3 seconds).

17. To give cardiopulmonary resuscitation to the newborn:
    - Place one hand under the baby's back.
    - With the tips of the index and middle fingers of the other hand, depress the midsternum about 1/2 to 3/4 inches.
    - Gently but forcibly do this at a rate of 80 to 100 compressions per minute (a little over one compression per second).
    - Give mouth-to-mouth resuscitation once after every 5 compressions.
    - Do not interrupt the compressions while doing the mouth-to-mouth breathing.

18. It is essential to squeeze the air from the bulb when using a bulb syringe to suction the newborn before inserting the syringe into the baby's mouth or nose because failure to do so could injure the baby's lungs.

19. To properly massage the woman's uterus after the baby is born, place one hand around the fundus of the uterus. Fingers should be deep into the abdomen behind the fundus; the thumbs should rest on the top of the fundus. Place the other hand on

ANSWERS 197

the mother's abdomen just above the pubic bone. This hand is used only to support the uterus. Do not massage or apply pressure with this hand. Massage the fundus of the uterus vigorously with a circular motion until it becomes firm. Never squeeze the uterus.

20. Signs that indicate the placenta has separated from the wall of the uterus are:
    - The umbilical cord advances approximately 3 or more inches farther out of the vagina.
    - A trickle or sudden spurt of blood flows from the vagina.
    - The uterus feels like a round ball and usually becomes more firm.

21. After the placenta has delivered, the uterus should feel like a firm, round mass below the navel and remain that way. If it does not feel like this, massage the uterus until it remains firm.

22. The uterus must be firm before the placenta is delivered, otherwise it could turn inside out causing very grave complications.

23. Five things to do if the woman is hemorrhaging are:
    - Massage the uterus until it feels firm.

198 ANSWERS

- If hemorrhage does not stop from massaging the uterus, place towels or clean cloths over the vagina and perineum.
- Cross the woman's legs tightly.
- Elevate the lower half of her body.
- Encourage the baby to nurse.
- Seek medical help immediately.

24. To properly cut the umbilical cord:

    - Place the baby on its side on a clean towel.
    - Wait until the cord has stopped pulsating.
    - Handle the cord carefully.
    - Use an antiseptic to clean the cord.
    - Tie the cord with a square knot approximately 4 to 6 inches from the baby's navel.
    - Leave a space of one to two inches and tie off again using a square knot.
    - Tie the knot slowly making sure the knot is tight.
    - Cut the cord between the two ties with a sterile instrument.
    - Check the end of the cord attached to the baby periodically after cutting for any signs of continued bleeding.

25. If there are signs of bleeding from the cord after it has been tied and cut, tie the cord again between the first tie and the belly button.

26. If any part other than the baby's head or buttocks presents, give emotional support and get medical help immediately.

27. If contractions are 2 minutes apart and birth is not occurring within 20 minutes, take the woman to the hospital without delay.

28. In a breech delivery, if the head does not deliver within 3 minutes after the body, insert 2 fingers gently into the baby's mouth and bend its chin down on the chest. With the other hand, apply firm pressure on the mother's abdomen. If the head still does not deliver, create and maintain an air passage to the baby's nose so it does not suffocate by placing two fingers into the vagina with the palm of your hand towards the baby's face. Place your fingers at each side of the baby's nose forming a "v." Press the wall of the vagina away from the baby's face with the back of your fingers.

29. Elevate the hips. Place her in knee-chest position and then on her side with hips elevated on pillow(s).

30. Do not handle the premature baby any more than is absolutely necessary. Remember to: (1) help baby breathe, (2) keep baby warm, (3) handle with care, and (4) prevent infection.

200 ANSWERS

31. A multiple birth may be expected if the woman's abdomen is unusually large before delivery and if it stays very large after the delivery of one baby.

32. Three complications that are more likely to occur when there is a multiple birth are: (1) the expulsion of the placenta may be more difficult; (2) there is a greater tendency for the mother to hemorrhage; (3) resuscitation efforts of the newborns are more likely.

33. Immediate care of the mother after delivery includes:

    - Checking frequently to be sure the uterus remains firm (if it relaxes massage until it is again firm).
    - Cleansing the vulva with a clean moist cloth or pouring warm, soapy water over the vaginal opening and rinsing with warm water.
    - If the perineum has been torn during delivery, treating it as an open wound by applying direct pressure to the bleeding area with a gauze pad or clean cloth.
    - Elevating the mother's hips and legs if bleeding is severe.
    - Covering the vaginal opening with a sanitary napkin or clean cotton cloth.

- Wiping the mother's face and hands with a damp cloth and drying with a clean towel.
- Keeping the mother warm.
- Giving the mother as much liquid as she desires, unless she is nauseous or for other reasons this is not advisable.
- Giving the mother emotional support.
- Letting the mother rest.

34. The baby's head must be supported whenever it is carried or lifted because it is larger and heavier than the rest of the body and the infant does not yet have control.

35. Signs of internal bleeding are: (1) rapid, weak pulse; (2) sudden drop in blood pressure; (3) skin pallor; (4) cold, clammy skin; (5) fainting or dizziness; (6) possible vomiting of blood; (7) if internal bleeding is slow and lasts for several hours, the patient shows apathy, lethargy, and confusion or restlessness.

36. If the baby is stillborn, it should be baptized, if appropriate. The mother should be given the option of seeing and holding her stillborn infant. Give emotional and psychological support to the mother. Wrap the baby in a sheet or blanket, attach identifying information, and transport to the hospital.

ADDRESSES AND TELEPHONE NUMBERS
DOCTORS

HOSPITALS

NOTES AND COMMENTS

982(1C2240H)